The Age of Agony

GUY WILLIAMS

The Age of Agony

THE ART OF HEALING

C 1700–1800

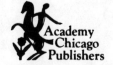

Academy
Chicago
Publishers

Published in 1986 by

Academy Chicago Publishers
425 N. Michigan Avenue
Chicago, Illinois 60611

Copyright © 1975 by Guy Williams

Printed and bound in the USA

Library of Congress Cataloging-in-Publication Data
Williams, Guy R.
    The age of agony.

    Reprint. Originally published: London, Constable, 1975.
    Bibliography: p.
    Includes index.
    1. Medicine—History—18th century. I. Title. [DNLM: 1. History
    of Medicine, 18th Cent. WZ 56 W723a 1975a]
R148.W54   1986   610'.941   85-30620
ISBN 0-89733-202-4
ISBN 0-89733-203-2 (pbk.)

For Basil and Bronwen Heaton

Contents

Illustrations

Preface

This book deals with the art of healing as it was practised, all too tragically, during the eighteenth century. It has not been possible, though, to begin precisely at the year AD 1700, and to finish equally exactly with the year in which the nineteenth century dawned. Too much that happened in the period under review can only be satisfactorily explained if some account is given of events that took place a century or more earlier. And, too many decisions that were made between 1700 and 1800 can only be called wise, or foolish, if the consequences of those decisions—seen after a suitably long interval of time—are carefully examined.

Many people have helped with the preparation of this book. I am especially grateful to Mr Benjamin Glazebrook, who first suggested that this might be a fascinating field of research. My thanks are due, too, to Miss Kerling, Archivist of St Bartholomew's Hospital, London, who has allowed me to inspect many of the historically invaluable documents in her care; Mr J H E Orde, Archivist of Guy's Hospital, who has also been enormously helpful; Mr R W Sharpington, Public Relations Officer of St Thomas's Hospital, who has provided much indispensable information; the Librarian and staff of the Wellcome Institute of the History of Medicine who have gone to much trouble to further my enquiries; the staff of the East Sheen branch of the Richmond Libraries, who have kindly obtained books for me—many of them, rare—from all parts of this country; and Miss Barbara Harris, who has patiently and accurately acted as typist and checker.

The Age of Agony

. . . Physicians of the utmost fame
Were called at once; but when they came
They answered, as they took their fees,
'There is no cure for this disease . . .'

HILAIRE BELLOC, 1870–1953

The English novelist E M Forster lived until 1970. When he was a little boy, Forster received from his great-aunt Marianne Thornton a letter in which, to entertain her young relative, the old lady described some of the notable events that she, when she herself was a child, had witnessed. As a very small girl, she said, she had been taken to Westminster to see King George III open a parliament. The king, though very ill, had insisted on going to meet his faithful Lords and Commons. Old Miss Thornton recalled:

> . . . There he was sitting on his throne with his king's crown on, his robes scarlet, velvet and ermine, held his speech written out for him just what he had to say. But Oh dear he stood up and made a bow and began 'My Lords and Peacocks'. The people who were not fond of him laughed, the people who did love him cried, and he went back to be no longer a King and his eldest son reigned in his stead and Regent Street was named after him . . .'

King George III succeeded to the throne of England, Scotland, Ireland and certain lands overseas in 1760. Put like that, the eighteenth century does not seem, in terms of years, at all distant.

Though comparatively near to us in time, the eighteenth century must have been, in many respects, as unlike our own as our own is perceptively different from the Great Ice Age. Both the

I

eighteenth century and the Great Ice Age were, beyond argument, for most people thoroughly unpleasant periods in which to exist.

If someone living today could be translated by a magician into the eighteenth century, he would probably appreciate the exquisite manners of the relatively few rich people about, and he might covet their unrivalled furniture—straight from Mr Chippendale's workshops, possibly—and their beautiful silver, porcelain and glass. Probably, he would enjoy the elegant music to which his new acquaintances danced their leisurely measures. But he would also find that he was immediately affected by certain particular discomforts, many of which he would never have experienced before. He would never be able to enjoy town life, for instance, without being constantly afflicted by the most disgusting smells. Wherever he was, he would be likely to itch so badly that he might wonder if the Devil himself were trying out on him some new and especially effective torments. Worst possibly of all, he would find that pain—excruciating and undiminishing pain, for which he could get no effective remedy or alleviation—was one of the inescapable liabilities of human existence.

Do we realize sufficiently what we have escaped by being alive in the twentieth, not the eighteenth, century? The following pages will tell.

2

Blood to Let

. . . Wonderful little, when all is said,
Wonderful little our fathers knew.
Half their remedies cured you dead—
Most of their teaching was quite untrue . . .

RUDYARD KIPLING, 1865–1936

It is fairly easy to see now, even from this relatively short distance of time, why the arts of healing developed so slowly during the eighteenth century. For one thing, the social and political conditions that prevailed at the time were wholly unfavourable for the necessary research. And, in certain other respects, the dice were heavily loaded against the doctors.

There was, to start with, an almost total lack of concern for public and personal hygiene. That, by itself, would have made it almost impossible for anyone to effect any real progress in medical and surgical affairs.

As late as March 1853, a contributor to *The Builder* magazine was able to write:

> . . . Let us look at the valley of the Fleet, Clerkenwell. Within
> the liberties of the City . . . this most abominable of rivers has
> been hidden from the sight . . .

A little to the north of the new street that had been built over the Fleet River—it was a continuation of the present-day Farringdon Street—there was a wooden hoarding running up for some distance. A tall man could peep over this, said the writer, and could see and hear the Fleet rolling in an unwholesome stream. A more enterprising traveller who, anxious to get an anecdote or two of the ancient stream, followed its apparent course in a northward direction would find that the Fleet, having appeared to the

3

light of day, passed for several hundred yards through the dense population. If, here, he dived down various courts and, by the favour of individuals, peeped out of dilapidated windows over-looking the Fleet in hopes of discovering the end of its polluted course, he would find that the stream was the sewer for the refuse of a population of more than half a million persons:

> ... Few men could view the blackness and hear the rolling of the Fleet, not to mention its effect on the other senses, without feeling pity for all residing near it ...

That was in 1853. In 1753 the Fleet sewer was uncovered right to where its load of sludge, rubbish and dead bodies oozed nauseatingly into the Thames.

Drunkenness, in the eighteenth century, was a condition that was accepted as inevitable almost as universally as dirtiness was tolerated.

In 1721, when the orgy of spirit drinking which was to last in the English capital for more than thirty years had just begun, the justices of the City of Westminster suggested that 'the principal cause of the increase of our poor and all the vice and debauchery among the inferior sort of people, as well as of the felonies and other disorders committed in and about this town' was the great increase of alehouses and spirit shops. There was no part of the town where the numbers of these places did not daily increase, said the justices, though they were so numerous already that in some of the larger parishes every tenth house at least sold 'one sort or another of those liquors by retail'. By 1743, every sixth house in the metropolis was believed to be a dram shop. Men, women and children dropped, dead drunk, in the street and lay, inert and helpless, where they had fallen.

In his *Enquiry*, published in 1751, Henry Fielding, the Bow Street magistrate, reported that:

> ... Should the drinking this poison be continued in its present height during the next twenty years, there will be by that time few of the common people left to drink it ... Gin is the principal sustenance (if it may be so called) of more than a hundred thousand people in the metropolis ... The intoxicat-

ing draught itself disqualifies them from any honest means to acquire it, at the same time that it removes sense of fear and shame and emboldens them to commit every wicked and desperate enterprise . . .

The gin cellars of London, during the eighteenth century, were more sordid than the sleaziest Soho dives of the present day. In these dank and unwholesome basements, drunken people sat in rows on filthy straw, or leaned in a comatose state against the louse-infested walls until they had sobered up sufficiently to be able to begin lowering the local fire-water all over again. Not much money was needed, in those days, for an adult to get hopelessly drunk, for spirits were not then heavily taxed as they are today. To get the small amount required—said Henry Fielding's brother John, in his *Account of the Police*, published in 1758—parents would send their syphilis-scarred children out begging on the streets.

It is impossible to review, even briefly, the drunkenness that prevailed in the eighteenth century without considering the brutalities of the time, for these two evils—intoxication and savagery—usually went hand in hand, the one being largely stimulated by the other.

Early in August 1732—according to the *Gentleman's Magazine*—a Mrs Eleanor Beare was brought to trial at Derby, which was then not a very large English country town.

Mrs Beare was indicted, in the first instance, 'for endeavouring to persuade one Nicholas Wilson to poison his wife, and for giving him poison to that end'. On a second indictment, Mrs Beare was required to answer for a 'Misdemeanour, in destroying the Foetus in the Womb of *Grace Belfort*, by putting an iron Instrument up into her Body, and thereby causing her to miscarry'.

Counsel for His Majesty the King, rising in all his legal glory in the provincial sessions, said that Mrs Beare had done something so shocking that he could not well display the nature of her crime to the court, but would have to leave it to the evidence. It was 'cruel and barbarous to the last degree'. After some unsupported and not very convincing chit-chat had been heard from, and about, one Nicholas Wilson, the girl named Grace Belfort was called to the witness box, and made this statement:

... I lived with the Prisoner as a Servant about ten Days, but was not hired, and was off and on with her about fourteen Weeks: When I had been with her a few Days there came Company into the House, and made me drink Ale and Brandy (which I was not used to drink) and it overcame me; my Mistress sent me into the Stable to give Hay to some Horses, but I was not capable of doing it, so laid me down in the Stables, and there came to me one *Ch——r*, a young Man that was drinking in the House, and after some Time I feared I was with Child by *Ch——r*, upon that my Mistress asked me if I was with Child, I told her I thought I was; Then she said if I could get 30 Shillings from *Ch——r*, she would clear me from the Child, without giving me Physick. A little Time after, some Company gave me Cyder and Brandy, my Mistress and I were both full of Liquor, and when the Company was gone, we could scarce get upstairs, but we did get up; then I laid me on the Bed, and my Mistress brought a kind of an Instrument, I took it to be like an Iron Skewer, and she put it up into my Body a great Way, and hurt me.

COURT: What followed upon that?

EVIDENCE: Some Blood came from me.

COURT: Did you miscarry after that?

EVIDENCE: The next Day after I went to *Allestree*, where I had a miscarriage.

COURT: What did the Prisoner do after this?

EVIDENCE: She told me the Job was done ...

The case turned out badly for Mrs Beare. She was found guilty, ordered to stand in the pillory on the next two market days, and to suffer close confinement for three years. The *Gentleman's Magazine* had a reporter present on 18 August 1732 when the unfortunate abortionist was exposed to the fury of the mob, for the first time, in the Derby market square:

... To which Place she was attended by several of the Sherif's Officers; notwithstanding which, the Populace, to shew their Resentment of the horrible Crimes wherewith she had been charged, and the little Remorse she has shewn since her Commitment, gave her no Quarter, but threw such quantities of Eggs, Turnips, Etc that it was thought she would hardly have escaped with her Life: She disengaged herself from the Pillory before the Time of her standing was expired, and jump'd among the Crowd, whence she was with Difficulty carried back to Prison . . .

On 25 August 1732, Mrs Beare was made to stand in the pillory again:

. . . As soon as she mounted she kneel'd down and beg'd Mercy of the outragious Mob. The Officers finding it difficult to get her Head thro' the Hole, pull'd off her Head-Dress, and found a large Pewter Plate beat out fit for her Head, which was thrown amongst the People; and as soon as she was fixed, such Showers of Eggs, Turnips, Potatoes, Etc were thrown, that it was expected she wou'd not have been taken down alive. She lost a great deal of Blood, which running down the Pillory, a little appeased their Fury. Those who saw her afterwards in the Gaol, said, she was such an Object as was not fit to be look'd on . . .

With barbaric occasions of that sort occurring frequently in almost every town, almost to the end of the eighteenth century, it is hardly surprising that the equally barbaric forms of treatment dispensed by the physicians and surgeons of the period were accepted without any significant protest.

Why, one could ask, were those forms of treatment generally so crude and inhumane?

The question is easily answered. The sciences of medicine and surgery were, as we have said, seriously retarded. They had remained in a comparatively primitive state because no one had managed, so far, to establish their basic principles. That was to come, at a relatively late moment in time. During most of the eighteenth century, theories based on the wildest guesswork were still being believed without being tested by any form of scientific examination, and some of the most ludicrous of those fallacies were still being widely accepted as true, long after their improbabilities should have been obvious to all.

There was Hippocrates' humoral pathology, for instance. This ancient doctrine, which attributed all disease to disorders of the 'humours' or nervous fluids of the body, ought to have been entirely discredited by the beginning of the eighteenth century, yet there were few, if any, important medical men alive at that time who did not subscribe, still, to this early but erroneous concept.

One of the most important of them all was Georg Ernst Stahl. Stahl—born in Ansbach, Bavaria, in 1660—dabbled as a young man in magic and alchemy. Having graduated in medicine at the University of Jena, he became, in 1687, court physician to the King of Prussia. Stahl was largely responsible for the theory that matter, when burning, gave off a substance that he called 'phlogiston', the material left being changed to 'calx'—a false theory that delayed the progress of the study of chemistry for nearly a century. He saw the human body as a kind of shrine which was inhabited by the 'anima'—the life force or immortal soul. If the soul started to misdirect its activities, taught Stahl, the body's vital functions would be disturbed. He and those of his followers who based their diagnoses and treatments on his incorrect ideas were fond of recommending 'secret' remedies which, they said, had a suggestive effect on the soul.

Stahl had a great rival—Friedrich Hofmann, of Halle. Hofmann, born in the same year as Stahl, despised his famous contemporary's 'anima' concept and he based his own system of medicine more exactly on the humours or nervous fluids described by Hippocrates more than two thousand years before. These fluids—which, according to Hofmann, were secreted by the brain—flowed from there in an ether-like way to various parts of the body. If the fluids flowed too freely to any one part, said Hofmann, an acute trouble that he called a 'spasm' would result. If they failed to flow freely enough, a chronic condition that he called 'atony' would appear. To treat a spasm, taught Hofmann, the physician should apply relaxing substances and fluids which would act as sedatives or soothers. To treat an atonic condition, he should apply some stimulant or irritant such as camphor, quinine or ether. The humours of the body would thus be kept in a controlled state of motion. This, said Hofmann, was necessary for the preservation of perfect health.

Most sympathetic, perhaps, of all the eighteenth-century

8

medical theorizers and system-makers was William Cullen, who was born at Hamilton, in Lanarkshire, Scotland, in 1710. One of the most prodigious of them was Cullen's pupil John Brown, who was born at a village in the parish of Buncle, in Berwickshire, exactly a quarter of a century later.

Cullen's father was factor to the Duke of Hamilton. At an early age, the boy was sent to Glasgow University, where he became the pupil of an earnest medical man named Paisley. Paisley's good medical library and studious habits are known to have had a profound influence on Cullen.

When he was nineteen, Cullen went to London and got a job as a surgeon on a merchant ship that was commanded by a relative. On his first journey abroad, the young man went to the West Indies and stayed for six months at Portobello. When he returned to London, he worked for some time as an assistant to an apothecary in Henrietta Street, Covent Garden. In what should have been his leisure hours, Cullen assiduously continued his studies.

Then his father and his eldest brother died suddenly, and Cullen felt obliged to return to Scotland to help to look after, and to earn money for, his younger brothers and sisters. After two years of doing that, he was fortunate enough to inherit a small legacy, which enabled him to go to the Edinburgh Medical School to study under the celebrated Alexander Monro (the first of three great Edinburgh doctors of that name). Cullen graduated as Doctor of Medicine in 1740 and began to practise. In 1751, he became Professor of Medicine at Glasgow University and in 1755 he was elected Joint Professor of Chemistry at Edinburgh.

Each morning, after he had received that appointment at Edinburgh, Cullen would rise before seven and would usually dictate to a hired clerk until nine. At ten, he would begin his visits to his patients, proceeding in a sedan chair through the narrow closes and winding alleys of that ancient city. When he had been doing this for two years, and had built up an extensive practice, he began to give clinical lectures, in the afternoons, in the Infirmary.

In his lectures, Cullen sought to disillusion all the old-fashioned practitioners who still believed in Hippocrates' and Friedrich Hofmann's 'humours'. Having spent a lot of time surveying the damage that diseases did to the solid structures of the body, the Edinburgh man was convinced that Hofmann's doctrine, in which the emphasis was laid on fluids, real or imaginary, was based on false premises and could only lead to fatal results. In the study of solids, not fluids, said Cullen, lay the future of healing. Life itself, he taught, was a function of nervous energy.

Cullen's lectures soon became renowned and attracted more and more people—possibly because he delivered them in English, instead of the Latin that had formerly been thought obligatory for medical lessons. One of his pupils recorded that Cullen's students were ardently attached to him because 'he was cordially attentive to all their interests, admitted them freely to his house, conversed with them on the most familiar terms, solved their doubts and difficulties, gave them the use of his library, and in every respect treated them with the affection of a friend and the regard of a parent'. He is known to have assisted, financially, so many impoverished students that he remained, himself, a relatively poor man.

Into this happy and harmonious nest came that egregious and disturbing cuckoo, the brilliant John Brown.

By the age of thirteen, Brown had been made a pupil-teacher in the local school in his native Berwickshire. He had a fantastically retentive memory. One of the boys he taught recalled that Brown could go through two pages of Cicero with a class, after which he would close the book and repeat the whole passage word for word, without making a single mistake. The country folk, a little intimidated by his erudition, believed that Brown could 'raise the devil' whenever he wished for Auld Nick's company.

When he was twenty-four, this clever young man decided to enter the medical profession. His fame had spread, and he was allowed by Alexander Monro and one or two other Edinburgh professors to attend their lectures free. He soon started to give private lessons to his fellow students—helping, when they needed aid with their Latin, to prepare them for their examinations. The medical students at that time were as convivial as their means allowed, and often more so, and before long Brown was drinking heavily and more or less constantly in debt.

By his intellectual brilliance, however, he attracted the favourable attention of William Cullen, and the older man soon took the younger one into his employment—first, as a general tutor to the Cullen children; later, as a kind of assistant to himself.

There were, in Brown's nature, other weaknesses besides his addiction to alcohol and his inability to manage his personal finances with any success.

He was prone, for instance, to seek the company of those who were either younger or less gifted than himself, and he enjoyed earning the admiration of his acolytes by pouring scorn on the beliefs and practices of all medical men who were senior to, and probably wiser than, themselves. Even Cullen, who had so effectively befriended Brown, did not escape the younger man's contempt.

By 1778 Brown had fallen out with most of the Edinburgh professors, including Monro and Cullen, and he made matters worse by giving a series of public lectures on 'The Practice of Physic'. In these lectures, Brown tried to show the errors in all previous systems of medicine; Cullen's 'nervous energy' theories earned Brown's particularly virulent contempt.

In his lectures, and in his writings, Brown propounded the wholly original idea that the quality or principle on which life depended could be defined as 'excitability'. He divided the exciting powers, or 'stimuli', into two classes. These were the *external stimuli*, which included heat, diet, and other substances taken into the stomach; the blood, the fluids secreted from the blood, and air: and the *internal stimuli*, which included muscular contraction, sense and perception, and the energy of the brain in thinking and in exciting passion and emotion.

If the exciting powers are withdrawn, Brown claimed, death will inevitably follow. Good health, he said, depends on the maintenance of a state of moderate excitability. Disease results when that happy equilibrium is broken down—by some local or general increase or decrease of excitability. Accordingly, he divided diseases into two main groups: *sthenic diseases*, which occur when excitability is increased, and *asthonic diseases*, which occur when excitability is lessened.

Therapy, according to Brown's system, was quite straightforward. If the patient were suffering from a sthenic disease, the physician should prescribe a sedative. If he, or she, were suffering from an asthonic disease, the physician should prescribe a stimulant. What could be simpler, as a formula for universal well-being?

Before he had been lecturing and writing for long, Brown found that he was able to attract a crowd of supporters—they called themselves 'Brunonians'. Many of the Brunonians were as excitable (and as argumentative, and as pugnacious) as Brown himself. Ranged against the Brunonians there were the 'Cullenians'—followers of Brown's more placid and conservative mentor —who were equally pigheaded. The rival mobs were as vociferous as they were stubborn—not so very unlike the partisan crowds that pay to watch Scottish football matches today.

For eight years, then, Brown carried on his campaign against the Edinburgh professors and the general body of medical practitioners in the city. He had, we know, what we would call today a 'charismatic personality'. We can get a glimpse of him at his most dynamic from the pages of his biographer Thomas Beddoes:

> ... His voice was in general hoarse and rather croaking ...
> Before he began his lecture, he would take 40 or 50 drops of laudanum in a glass of whisky, repeating the dose four or five times during the lecture. Between the effects of these stimulants and voluntary exertion, he soon waxed warm, and by degrees his imagination was exalted into phrenzy ...

Laudanum—a hallucinatory drug derived from the opium poppy —and whisky, those were Brown's favourite remedies. Soon, he became addicted to both. His health suffered in consequence. Fewer and fewer patients came to him, and his public lectures attracted steadily diminishing audiences. At last he was lodged in prison for debt. Just a few loyal students continued to attend him there, for tuition. (A truly romantic gesture, typical of all supporters of hopelessly lost causes.)

After that, in 1786, Brown left Edinburgh and moved with his family to London, establishing himself in a house in Golden Square. He continued to give lessons, and attempted to build up some sort of a practice, but debts once more overtook him and he was obliged to take up residence once more in confinement—on this occasion, in the King's Bench Prison. Writing alone seemed to offer him any chance of escaping from the clutches of his creditors, and when a publisher offered him £500 to produce a treatise on the gout, it seemed as if his fortunes might be about to be restored. Perhaps—we do not know this for certain, but it is not unlikely—Brown celebrated this improvement in his prospects a little too liberally. He died unexpectedly, we know, during one night, less than two years after he arrived in the capital, having taken too powerful a dose of laudanum on retiring.

John Brown's ideas (like his namesake's soul) went marching on. Brown's *Elementa Medicinae*, written in flawless Latin, and first published in Edinburgh in 1780, was reprinted at Milan in 1792 and at Hildburghausen in 1794. The English version was republished at Philadelphia in 1790 by the famous American Doctor Benjamin Rush (it became the lonely frontiersman's medical bible); and translations were published in Denmark, France, Germany and Italy. An exposition of the Brunonian system with all the relevant literature was published in two volumes by Girtanner at Göttingen in 1799. As late as 1802, the University of Göttingen was so convulsed by controversy on the merits and demerits of the Brunonian system that contending factions of students in enormous numbers, aided by their professors, met in combat in the streets on two successive days and had to be dispersed by a troop of Hanoverian cavalry. Brown's therapeutic recommendations, which caused so much misuse of opium and alcohol, have been said to have destroyed more people than the French Revolution and the Napoleonic Wars combined.

Whichever school of thought they favoured—Stahl's or Hofmann's, Cullen's or Brown's—almost all medical men of the eighteenth century relied for their 'cures' principally on such drastic processes as the artificial raising of blisters, purging, the administration of toxic drugs, the inducement of vomiting, and blood-letting. Of these, the last was by far the most frequently used form of treatment.

The idea that a sick person could be relieved by the removal of some of the blood from his or her body was an ancient one. 'Let out the blood, let out the disease' was the basic principle of this dangerously ill-conceived practice. For hundreds of years, it was the most popular form of treatment for any serious illness. During the eighteenth century, the urge to draw blood became almost a frenzy. As late as 1781, William Moss, a Liverpool surgeon, was writing in his *Essay on the Management and Nursing of Children in the Earlier Periods of Infancy*:

> ... Bleeding is a remedy much to be depended on when the symptoms of heat, fever, drowsiness and startings are urgent: it is commonly done to children by means of leeches, which may be applied to the foot or heel, and may be repeated every day or every other day while these symptoms continue with any degree of severity. Two leeches may be applied at one time to a child about three months old, and three to one of five or six months ...

Treatment by leeches was so prevalent in the early days of St George's Hospital, London, that—according to one item in the governors' minutes—'Mr Butler and Mr Hunter are requested to send to the Hospital every second Tuesday the price of leeches and state at what price they will supply the institution during the ensuing fortnight.'

When leeches were not used, blood-letting was carried out, normally by opening a superficial vein—usually a vein in the arm; sometimes a vein in the hand.

The operation was usually performed by a barber or barber-surgeon, acting under a physician's or apothecary's instructions. The sign still seen outside some men's hairdresser's shops evolved quite naturally from the trade sign of the barber-surgeon, which was an arm bound by a tourniquet and holding a bowl. (The bowl served a double purpose. It was used for making lather for shaving, on some occasions, and for catching blood on others.) In the modern version of this sign the pole represents the arm, the red stripes painted on it represent the patient's bloody flesh, the white stripes represent the tourniquet and the globe—if there is one—has taken the place of the dish.

Two items of equipment used for blood-letting in the eighteenth century still survive in reasonably large numbers and can still, in fact, be collected. *Bleeding bowls* made of tin-glazed earthenware, pewter, silver and other materials are found—many of them, with graduation lines marked on the inside which were intended to show, at a glance, how many ounces of blood had been drawn from the patient. The small pocket *lancets* taken by eighteenth-century physicians on their rounds were often carried in attractive cases made of silver, shagreen, tortoiseshell, or some other relatively expensive material.

Spring-operated 'fleans' or 'schnappers', invented for blood-letters by a German surgeon during the late seventeenth century, can still be studied in some museums. The 'scarificator'—developed a little later—was a brass or silver box that contained six to twelve short curved blades, controlled by a spring and a trigger. When the case was pressed against the patient's skin, and the trigger was pulled, the blades would be released simultaneously, making the required incisions. A warmed cup would then be placed over the spot to draw out the blood.

We know, now, exactly what blood-letting must have been like for the patient, because we can study (if we care to) an instruction manual for barbers—the *Prattica Nova, di tutto quello ch'al Barbiero s'appartrene* by Cintio D'Amato, first published in Venice in 1669, the principles of which were still being followed a hundred years later. When D'Amato dealt with the correct method of making incisions in the veins of the hand, he recommended that two veins only should be used. The first, which comes down from the head, should be opened, he said, only where it joins the trunk vein above the thumb, or at the elbow. The second—the *salvatelle* —which ended according to his observations between the little finger and the ring finger should be tapped in the left hand for affections of the spleen and in the right for affections of the liver.

To bleed this vein well, D'Amato advised, it was essential for the attending barber to prepare hot water in which the patient's hand could be placed, so that the heat would swell the vein and make it more prominent. In a short time, the location of the vein could be traced by gentle rubbing with the left thumb. If the vein's location could not be positively discovered, two fingers could be bled, well away from the place.

An important part in the bleeding operation was played by the ligature bandage or tourniquet. When thin persons were being bled, recommended D'Amato, this ought not to be too tight because of the pain it caused, and because thin people were more sensitive than fat. Fat people could have the ligature tied very tightly, he said, and the bandage could be located farther away from the site of the incision so that the vein should not be shut off.

Having located the vein, and having tied the ligature, the barber, following D'Amato's instructions, would take the patient's hand in a linen napkin, holding it firmly so that there would be no possibility of the hand being freed from his grip. Then, he would hold the patient's finger and would stretch it somewhat while, with his lancet, he pierced the vein longitudinally. After he had made this incision, the barber would dip the patient's hand in hot water again, to make the blood flow more freely, 'heat having the property of opening the vein and liquefying the blood'. When sufficient blood had been drawn off, the wound would be bound up, but not so tightly that 'coarse and impure blood' could not continue to escape.

In 1735 the Breton Alain-Réné Le Sage published the last two volumes of his picaresque novel, *Gil Blas of Santillane*. At one stage of his adventures, Le Sage's hero is able to study a Doctor Sangrado, whose methods of bleeding and 'drenching' were, if a little exaggerated, still fairly typical of those fashionable at that stage of the eighteenth century:

. . . I stayed for three months with the Canon Sedillo [recounts Gil Blas] and lost little sleep during that time.

At the end of the three months, my employer became ill. He caught a fever, and it inflamed his gout. For the first time in his very long life he sent for a physician. Doctor Sangrado was the man he called in—the 'Hippocrates of Valladolid'. Dame Jacintha [the Canon's housekeeper] suggested that a lawyer should be sent for, first, but the patient thought that there was time enough for that, and he was still strong enough to get his own way—in certain directions.

So, I went to fetch Doctor Sangrado, and brought him back with me. He was, I found, a tall, sallow, shrunken executioner, who had been doing Fates' deadly work for them for at least forty years. This learned forerunner of the undertaker looked just right for his job. He weighed every word carefully, before letting it fall, and he used lofty medical terms that could hardly fail to impress the uninitiated. He argued for the sake of arguing, and he expounded, as gospel, theories that had never been heard on earth before.

After he had studied my master's symptoms carefully for some time, Doctor Sangrado began a solemn medical lecture:

'What we have to do here, Gentlemen, is to unblock a perspiratory system that has become improperly ... er ... er ... *blocked up*. Ordinary doctors, asked to deal with a case like this, would probably prescribe the usual dreary old salines, diuretics, volatile salts, and sulphur and mercury ... Could any remedies be more *deadly* than these? ... My methods are simpler and much more effective' ... [To the patient] 'What is your usual diet?'

'My usual diet? I live on soups, mostly,' replied the Canon. 'And I eat a great deal of broth.'

'Soups and broth!' exclaimed the doctor, horrified. 'Goodness! No wonder you're ill! High living, of that kind, is like a bait charged with poison. It is a deadly trap set for self-indulgent people, to shorten their lives. We must stop giving way to our appetites—the more insipid food and drink are, the better they are for us ... Our veins aren't filled with broth, are they? Well then, we must only take in the kind of nourishment that will mingle with the particles of our blood. You drink wine, I suppose?'

'I do,' said the Canon. 'But watered down.'

'Oh, finely watered down, I dare say!' snapped the doctor. 'This is the height of intemperance! A terrible diet! You ought to have died years ago! How old are you?'

'I am in my sixty-ninth year,' answered the Canon.

'I thought as much!' said the doctor. 'Self-indulgent people always grow old before their time! You ought to have drunk clear water only, all your life, and you should have stuck to good plain food like boiled apples. If you had done that, you wouldn't be suffering so terribly with gout, now, and your limbs would still be functioning properly ... But, don't worry! I'll soon have you running about again, as long as you do exactly as I tell you.' The Canon promised to be a perfect patient.

Doctor Sangrado then sent me to fetch a barber-surgeon of his own choosing, and this man took from the Canon six good bowls full of blood, by way of a start, to relieve the obstinate blockage, Doctor Sangrado then said to the barber-surgeon: 'Mr Onez! You will please repeat the operation in three hours' time, removing the same amount of blood as you have just now, and tomorrow you will take as much again. It is quite wrong to suppose that blood has any useful function to perform in the human system—the quicker you can draw it off the better. A sick man has nothing else to do but to lie down quietly and keep alive. He doesn't need blood . . . He doesn't need blood, any more than a man asleep and dreaming needs blood . . . In both instances, life consists merely of "pulsation" and "respiration". Blood is unnecessary for these . . .'

When the doctor had prescribed these repeated and copious blood-lettings, he ordered that the patient should be given frequent and equally copious drenches of warm water at very short intervals. The administration of water in sufficient quantities was (he said) the basis of all healing.

Having made that authoritative pronouncement, Doctor Sangrado took his leave, telling Dame Jacintha, and me, with a confident air, that he would guarantee the patient's survival, as long as his instructions were properly followed.

Dame Jacintha was, secretly, horrified by these new-fangled medical techniques, but she was no match for the cool professional authority of Doctor Sangrado. So, she and I put the kettles urgently on the fire, and as soon as the water was warm enough we started to pour two or three pints of it down the patient's throat, as quickly as he could swallow. An hour later, we gave him another drench. We repeated the treatment time and time again, on each occasion pouring a regular cloudburst of clean warm water into the poor old Canon's stomach. As fast as we put in the water, the barber-surgeon drew off the blood. Between us, we brought the poor old Canon to death's door in less than forty-eight hours.

When the worthy old clergyman was about to expire, I tried to drink his health with a large glass of the new liquid refreshment with which he was being so liberally plied. 'Stop this, Gil Blas!' I heard him plead faintly. 'Don't give me any more, my friend. Death will come for me as soon as he pleases, however much water I have . . . And, I've scarcely got a drop of blood left in my veins, but I feel no better . . . In fact, I could hardly feel worse . . . The cleverest doctor in the world can do nothing to help us, when our time is up. Fetch a solicitor, will you? I want to make my will.'

When I heard the old man say these propitious words, I pretended to be sad. Hiding my eagerness to get off to the lawyer's, I answered: 'Don't give up yet, Sir! You're not as low as all that! You may get better, yet . . . '

'No! No!' he interrupted me. 'I won't. It's all up with me. I can feel my gout moving round, and Death has got his chill hand on me. Hurry up, and do what I have asked you to do . . . '

I saw, clearly enough, that the old man was sinking fast. So, I left Dame Jacintha to look after him (she was more scared of his dying without making a will, even, than I was!) and I ran as quickly as I could to find a solicitor—any solicitor. 'Sir!' I said, to the first properly qualified lawyer I managed to locate. 'Canon Sedillo, my master, is approaching his end. He wants to put his affairs in order. Come quickly, will you? There's not a moment to be lost!'

The solicitor was a dapper little chap, who enjoyed his joke. 'Who is your doctor?' he asked. When I mentioned Doctor Sangrado's name, he put his hat and coat on immediately. 'For pity's sake!' he cried. 'Let's get going without wasting a minute. Doctor Sangrado finishes his patients off so quickly that we lawyers can hardly keep up with him. That chap kills half my clients before I can get them nicely signed and sealed.'

. . . So [Dame Jacintha] and I left the solicitor alone with our poor old master, and we retired into one of the side rooms. There, to our great surprise, we found the barber-surgeon, who had been sent in by Doctor Sangrado to carry out just one more (and certainly final) experiment. We took hold of this gory person. 'Stop, Master Martin!' cried the housekeeper. 'You can't go into His Reverence's rooms just now! He is having his Last Wishes put down on paper. You can bleed away to your heart's content once the will is safely signed and sealed!'

We were both dreadfully afraid, this pious lady and I, that the Canon might pass away with his will half completed, but luckily the document, so important to both of us, was satisfactorily drawn up. We saw the solicitor leave the Canon's room. The lawyer, finding me on the alert, clapped me on the shoulder and said with a wink 'Gil Blas has not been forgotten!'

I felt so happy when I heard those words—so happy that I vowed I would have the pleasure of praying for my kind master's soul after his death. I did not have to wait long for that melancholy event, either, for when the barber-surgeon had bled him once more the poor old man, quite worn out, gave up the ghost under the lancet. Just as the Canon was drawing his last breath, Doctor Sangrado appeared, and looked a little foolish in spite of the number of death-beds at which he had similarly acted as a spectator. Far from blaming his bleeding-and-drenching therapy for the Canon's swift demise, the doctor declared boldly as he strode away that the outcome of the case was due to the attendants being too sparing of the lancet, and too careful of their warm water. The medical executioner—I mean, the barber-surgeon—seeing that his usefulness was over, followed Doctor Sangrado . . .

It would be unfair to leave this brief introduction to the sad tale of eighteenth-century medicine and surgery without stressing the fact that there were a few isolated figures working, during that century, in a largely scientific and therefore progressive way.

There was Albrecht von Haller, for instance.

Von Haller, who was born in Berne, in Switzerland, in 1708, studied and taught for seventeen years at the newly-established University of Göttingen. During this time, he achieved fame through his prodigious industry as an anatomist, a botanist and a physiologist. In the course of his working life, von Haller wrote more than thirteen thousand scientific papers, many of which announced important new discoveries he had made and which are universally accepted as significant contributions to the sum of human knowledge.

Scotland gave the world two further prodigies—the brothers William and John Hunter.

William Hunter—born at East Kilbride, Lanarkshire, in 1718—was educated at Glasgow University. Having studied medicine for a time under William Cullen at Hamilton and at Edinburgh, he

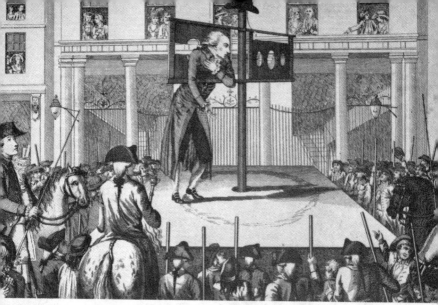

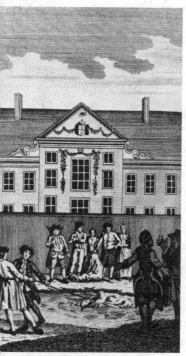

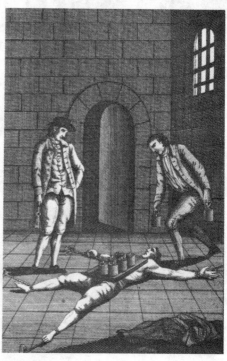

Top The Pillory, Mark Lane. *Lower left* The ducking of John Osborn and his wife on a charge of witchcraft. From The Old Bailey Chronicle Volume III. *Lower right* The punishment formerly inflicted on those who refused pleading to an indictment. Engraved for The Malefactors Register. Newgate Calendar Vol. I.

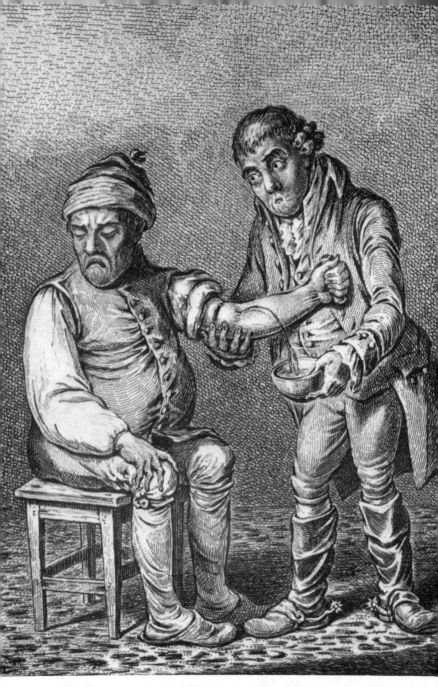

Breathing a vein, by Gillray 1804. Breathing was for the relief of apoplexy or blood pressure.

moved to London, where he soon earned a favourable reputation as an obstetrician, being appointed, in 1748, a surgeon-accoucheur at the Middlesex Hospital. In 1770 William Hunter took up residence in a house he had had built in Great Windmill Street (close to the present Piccadilly Circus). In this house, which contained dissecting-rooms and a lecture theatre, Hunter accommodated the encyclopaedic collection of anatomical, pathological and other scientific specimens he had been building up, many items from which can still be seen today at Glasgow University. Hunter—the first great teacher of anatomy in England—was a frugal liver of untiring industry who regularly gave lectures and demonstrations—lasting usually two hours—which were said to be both easy to understand, and profound.

John Hunter—born in 1728, the youngest of ten children—began his working life as a cabinet maker. When he was twenty, however, he was encouraged by his famous brother William to move to the English capital to act as his general assistant. John arrived in London about a fortnight before the beginning of his brother's autumnal course of lectures. In the following summer, he attended the lectures given by Sir William Cheselden at the Chelsea Military Hospital and watched the operations performed there by the celebrated surgeon. During the next winter the young man was thought to have acquired sufficient knowledge to be put in charge of his brother's 'practical anatomy' classes. Cheselden retired in 1751, upon which John Hunter became a surgeon's pupil at St Bartholomew's Hospital, where the renowned Percival Pott was one of the senior men. By 1756 Hunter had been appointed house surgeon to St George's Hospital at Hyde Park Corner. During the period of his connection with his brother's school, John Hunter solved the problem of the descent of the testes in the foetus, studied the nature of pus, explored the intricacies of the nasal and olfactory nerves that give us our sense of smell, and, with his brother, established the function and importance of the lymphatic glands in the animal—and therefore in the human—economy.

In the spring of 1759 John Hunter contracted some infection that gave him an inflammation of the lungs. Believing that he might be threatened with tuberculosis, he gave up his London work and went off as a staff surgeon in Hodgson and Keppel's expedition to Belleisle. In 1762 he was serving with the English armed forces on the frontier of Portugal. He retired on half pay early in 1763 and returned to England with a collection of about two hundred specimens of natural and diseased structures, all carefully preserved. (Many of John Hunter's invaluable acquisitions can be seen now, by the privileged, in the premises of the Royal College of Surgeons in Lincoln's Inn Fields, in London. Part of his collection was destroyed by German bombs in air raids in the Second World War.)

Once back in London, John Hunter took a house in Golden Square and started to practise, once again, as a civil surgeon. To eke out his inadequate pension, he taught anatomy and operative surgery to a private class. He devoted his few hours of leisure to the study of comparative anatomy, being given first refusal of the cadavers of all the animals that died in the menagerie at the Tower of London, and in various travelling zoological collections. At his house at Brompton, to the west of London, he assembled a lively stock of blackbirds, eagles, fishes, hedgehogs, toads and many other creatures that he kept for the purpose of observation and experiment. On two occasions, John Hunter's life was endangered by his 'pets'—once, when he had to struggle physically with a young bull, and to overcome it; and, later, when he courageously recaptured two leopards that had escaped and were savaging his dogs. Hunter collared the leopards and dragged them back to their dens.

In 1767 John Hunter ruptured his Achilles' tendon, and after this painful and crippling experience he performed on dogs several carefully devised experiments by which he was able to show that these essential but vulnerable parts of a body could be successfully re-united after being divided. These demonstrations of Hunter's laid the foundation for the modern practice of cutting through tendons ('tenotomy') for the relief of distorted and contracted joints.

In 1780 the Hunter brothers, under whose direct influence surgery had ceased to be merely a gory adjunct of the barber's trade and had been raised to the rank of a scientific profession, fell out, after John Hunter had read before the Royal Society a paper in which he implied that he had been the first person in the world to establish the nature of the circulation of the blood in the womb and its furnishings. Elder brother William who, five years previously, had described this exactly in his beautifully illustrated *Anatomy of the Gravid Uterus exhibited in Figures* then wrote to the Royal Society and claimed the honour for himself. 'Young' brother John countered this by sending a rejoinder to the Royal Society in which he tried to confirm what he had said before—he had made the discovery on a day in 1754 in a specimen injected by a Doctor Mackenzie, and had then told his brother what he had found. The total estrangement between the brothers that resulted from this correspondence lasted until the time of William's last illness, when John was allowed to visit his dying relative and, some say, to give him professional attention.

On the death of Percival Pott of St Bartholomew's Hospital in 1788, John Hunter was widely acclaimed as the First Surgeon in England. Hunter, himself, only lived to enjoy this eminence until 1793, but his influence was felt throughout the early nineteenth century, since nearly all the leading British physicians and surgeons of the period—and a great many American doctors too—had been, at some time, his pupils, and they had received from him a thorough training in anatomy, physiology, and the new science of surgical pathology which he had virtually created. 'When we make a discovery in pathology we only learn what we have overlooked in his [Hunter's] writings or forgotten in his lectures,' suggested Robert Adams, one of the founders of the Dublin School of Medicine, writing in 1818.

As the eighteenth century closed, a barely perceptible lightening of the gloom seemed to be announcing that the long awaited dawn of medical knowledge was approaching, thanks to a few dedicated and industrious men like Von Haller and the Hunters. To be able to appreciate fully the achievements of these men, we have to know how impenetrable was the darkness that came before that dawn.

3

The Perils of Pregnancy and Birth in the Eighteenth Century

Bliss was it in that dawn to be alive . . .

WILLIAM WORDSWORTH, 1770–1850

Doctor Charles White, who helped to found, in 1790, the Manchester Lying-In Hospital, wrote this harrowing description of the treatment normally given to maternity cases in the eighteenth century:

> . . . When the woman is in labour, she is often attended by a number of her friends in a small room, with a large fire, which, together with her own pains throw her into profuse sweats; by the heat of the chamber, and the breath of so many people, the whole air is rendered foul, and unfit for respiration; this is the case in all confined places, hospitals, jails, and small houses, inhabited by many families, where putrid fevers are apt to be generated, and proportionally the most so where there is the greatest want of free air. Putrid fevers thus generated are infectious, witness the black assize, as it is usually called.
>
> If the woman's pains are not strong enough, her friends are generally pouring into her large quantities of strong liquors, mixed with warm water, and if her pains are very strong, the same kind of remedy is made use of to support her. As soon as she is delivered, if she is a person in affluent circumstances, she is covered up close in bed with additional cloaths, the curtains are drawn round the bed, and pinned together, every crevice in the windows and door are stopped close, not excepting the key hole, the windows are guarded not only with shutters and curtains, but even with blankets, the more effectually to

exclude the fresh air, and the good woman is not suffered to put her arm, or even her nose out of bed, for fear of catching cold. She is constantly supplied out of the spout of a tea-pot with large quantities of warm liquors, to keep up perspiration and sweat, and her whole diet consists of them. She is confined to a horizontal posture for many days together, whereby both the stools and the lochia [matter evacuated from the uterus after a birth] are prevented from having a free exit. This happens not only from the posture of the patient, but also from the great relaxation brought on by warm liquors and the heat of the bed and room, which prevent the over extended abdominal muscles from speedily recovering their tone, whereby they are rendered unable to expel the contents of the abdomen, which lodging in the intestines many days become quite putrid . . .

From these sweaty, boozy and frequently hysteria-ridden lying-in rooms nearly all males were, at the beginning of the eighteenth century, rigidly excluded. By the end of the century, the male obstetrician had manoeuvred the female midwife into a secondary rôle. Childbirth had become, in consequence, a considerably less dangerous experience for both (or all) the parties principally concerned.

The entry of the male into the exclusively female labour room was due, to a great extent, to the members of the extraordinary Chamberlen family.

The Chamberlen story begins—at least as far as medical history is concerned—way back in 1569, when a small boy named Peter Chamberlen left France, with his father and mother, who were Huguenot refugees. (This is well before the period with which this book is supposed to deal, but the landing of the Chamberlens in Britain started a chain of events that was not to reach its conclusion until the eighteenth century was itself history.)

Three years later, Peter Chamberlen was living with his parents at Southampton. We know this, because he was old enough to sign documents concerning the birth and baptism of a new little brother. This later addition to the Chamberlen family was also named 'Peter', so, to avoid confusion, the two boys were afterwards referred to as 'Peter the Elder' and 'Peter the Younger' respectively.

By 1598 Peter the Elder was living in London and had been mentioned in the annals of the Barber-Surgeons' Company: 'His hood had been put on his shoulders and he had been admitted into the Liverie.' By 1603 he had worked up a good practice and could afford to pay the fines levied on him for ignoring the lectures the officers of the Livery required him to attend.

Peter the Elder's prosperity was due, at least in part, to the fact that he, before anyone else, had discovered how to make and use effective obstetric forceps. (The trick was to make two entirely separate blades that could be combined, and used like the blades of fire-tongs or dog-tongs *after* they had been humanely manoeuvred into position, one on each side of the baby.)

For several decades, Peter the Elder and the members of his family managed to keep this great secret successfully, and they managed equally successfully, to let all the world know that they *had* a secret. What could be more tantalizing and irresistible? So, the Chamberlens were called in, inevitably, to officiate at especially important births—as, for example, royal births—and, equally inevitably, their renown and self-importance earned them the hostility of more public-spirited medical men.

Peter the Elder was the first to suffer, when he became involved in the running battle that was being fought, at that time, between the physicians, the apothecaries and the barber-surgeons over the proper demarcation of the border-lines between their respective jobs—a prolonged squabble that foreshadowed some of the more squalid trade union disputes of the twentieth century. Having ventured to prescribe some liquids for a female patient to take internally, Peter the Elder found himself, in 1612, being accused by London's College of Physicians of 'not having confined himself strictly to the practice of surgery'—in other words, of having poached on somebody else's profitable territory. His activities were condemned and he was arrested and taken to the barbaric and nauseating prison at Newgate.

In such circumstances it helps to have friends in high places. Peter the Elder, having attended the Queen (Anne, wife of James I) in a difficult confinement, was comfortably situated. The Queen promptly instructed the Archbishop of Canterbury to intervene on her accoucheur's behalf, and Peter the Elder was (in obedience to the royal instructions) equally promptly released.

Four years later, Peter the Elder became involved, with his brother, in another *cause célèbre*. On this occasion the chief protagonists were the midwives 'in and about the City of London'. These good ladies—muscular, uneducated, and dangerously self-confident—banded together and took a petition to the Privy Council and the Attorney General, asking that they should be officially recognized and made into an Incorporated Society. The petition was supported by the Chamberlens and may, indeed, have been largely organized by them, for they saw in the scheme an opportunity for personal gain.

Opposition came from the members of the College of Physicians. While admitting that some way should be found for 'bettringe of the skill of the Midwives (who for the most part are very ygnorant)' the physicians did not think it right that the women should be allowed to form a self-governing body—which would largely be governed, the physicians suspected, by the hated Chamberlens.

So, the physicians came back with some counter-proposals. Up to that moment, the midwives had had to apply to the Bishop of London for permission to follow their trade. Why (said the physicians) should they not, instead, undergo a proper qualifying examination before they were licenced? The examination could easily be carried out by the President of the College and two or three of his senior associates. The suggestion so horrified the midwives that they forgot all about their plea for Incorporation. The physicians did not forget the part that the Chamberlens had played in the affair, however, and four years later, after a series of brushes with the College, Peter the Younger was forbidden to practise medicine altogether.

Peter the Younger's son comes into the story next. Born in 1601, he also was called Peter, but as this young man (unlike his father and his uncle) managed to obtain some indisputable medical qualifications, he is usually referred to as '*Doctor* Peter Chamberlen' when he is not given the royal-sounding title 'Peter the Third'.

Doctor Peter had, we know, an extraordinarily high opinion of himself. 'Some men have such an itch to quarrell' (said an anonymous contemporary of him) 'that rather than they will want objects they will fight with their owne shadowes, or make to themselves enemies of straw, that they may tear them to pieces and triumph in their ruine.' He was elected to a Fellowship of the College of Physicians on 29 March 1628 by a majority of votes, but the members did not approve of the frivolous and flashy clothes he affected, and the President was instructed to tell the successful candidate that his election would not be finally ratified unless he conformed to custom and adopted a decent and sober dress.

Hostilities between the College authorities and Doctor Peter broke out in deadly earnest in 1634, when another petition for the incorporation of midwives was presented by a Mrs Hester Shawe and a Mrs Whipp, who were both members of the sisterhood. On this occasion, the midwives were appealing for a charter in order to protect themselves against the Chamberlen family. Doctor Peter (so young, that he was 'no more bearded than any London midwife') had actually ordered the sisterhood to meet at his house once every month, so that he could licence the members individually to practise, if he saw fit. 'Out of an opinion of himself and his own ability in the Art of Midwifery,' was the verdict of the disgusted ladies. The smooth-faced young man had even dared to say that he would refuse to treat any woman in distress if her midwife had declined to conform to his will. Armed, as he was, with the secret obstetric forceps, he was making a meaningful threat. 'For aught as they could discern by his carriage,' said the midwives, 'Doctor Chamberlen would monopolize the whole practice among child-bearing women, being a young man, to the disparagement of all other Physicians and the Inslaving of your petitioners.' They claimed—probably with very good reason—that the young doctor often refused to attend poor people, who could not afford his fees. To the rich, they said, he denied his help until he had first made a bargain for some great reward. 'He wanted to get himself created Vicar-General of the Midwives in the City and Suburbs,' claimed his anonymous biographer. 'He would have a groate for every child born within his jurisdiction.'

The evidence given by the midwives and their friends was just what Doctor Peter's jealous rivals were looking for, and he was sharply rebuked. Frustrated in his attempt to organize the midwives to his own advantage, Doctor Peter embarked, next, on a series of enterprises intended to bring him more money and renown than even he, with the family secret, could hope to earn by practising as an obstetrician. He put to Parliament a vast scheme for providing 'Artificiall Bathes and Bath Stoves' for the use of the populace in all cities and towns in the kingdom. (The officials of the College of Physicians predictably opposed this scheme, saying that public baths, in the Greek and Roman States, had effeminated bodies and had debauched the manners of the people.) He published another scheme, a little crazier, for dissolving all debts. He devised a method of 'propelling ships and carriages by wind so that they would sail in a straight line whatever direction the wind came from'. Long before he died, at the spacious country seat he had purchased—Woodham Mortimer Hall, near Maldon in Essex—Doctor Peter had passed into a state of religious exaltation which bordered upon, and sometimes reached, lunacy.

The Chamberlen story features, next, Doctor Peter's son Doctor Hugh Chamberlen (often referred to, to distinguish him from his own son, as Doctor Hugh Chamberlen 'the Elder').

Doctor Hugh ('the Elder') was born about 1630, and as soon as he was old enough he followed the family calling. In 1673 he published his own translation of a book *Observations sur la Grossesse et l'Accouchement* written by the greatest living obstetrician, François Mauriceau, who happened to be working in France. For many decades, European midwives had been principally guided in their work by an instruction manual called *The Expert Midwife* by the Swiss Jacob Rueff that had been published in 1554. Mauriceau's book was much more scientific and up-to-date than Rueff's and contained less material that was likely to mislead. It was not offered to its English-speaking readers without certain reservations, though. In a preface specially prepared for the London edition by the translator, Doctor Hugh while complimenting the French author on the superiority of his work over that of previous writers, expressed his disapproval of two important features of Mauriceau's obstetric techniques—he did not think that delivery, in 'difficult' births, should be delayed, as the French accoucheur did; and he did not think much of the 'crotchets' or little hooks that the Frenchman recommended for use in natal emergencies. Doctor Hugh could not resist the temptation to include in his preface some personal sales talk, aimed at the home market:

> ... My Father, Brothers and my self (tho none else in Europe as I know) have, by God's Blessing and our Industry, attained to, and long practised a way to deliver women in this case without any prejudice to them or their infants; tho all others (being obliged, for want of such an expedient, to use the common way) do and must endanger if not destroy one or both with Hooks ...

By the Chamberlens' own 'manual operation', Doctor Hugh claimed, a labour could be dispatched with the least difficulty, with fewer pains, and more quickly, to the great advantage of, and without danger to, both woman and child:

> ... If therefore the use of Hooks by Physicians and Chirurgeons be condemned [he went on] without thereto necessitated through some monstrous Birth, we can much less approve of a Midwife's using them, as some here in England boast they do; which rash presumption in France, would call them in Question for their Lives ...

After that very persuasive puff for his own family's methods, Hugh Chamberlen must have felt that some apology should be made to his readers for his failure to publish the secret of extracting children from the womb without the use of hooks. Lamely, he explained:

> ... There being my Father and two Brothers living that practise this art, I cannot esteem it my own to dispose of, nor publish it without injury to them and I think I have not been unserviceable to my country altho I do but inform them that the forementioned three persons of our family and my self can serve them in these extremities with greater safety than others ...

Doctor Hugh gave the name *The Accomplisht Midwife* to his version of Mauriceau's great work. It was an immediate best seller. (It netted for Doctor Hugh as much as £30,000 per year, according to Mauriceau's possibly prejudiced estimate.) Until quite late in the eighteenth century it was by far the most popular text book with all who practised midwifery in Britain and America. It brought the Chamberlens more high-class—and therefore highly profitable—obstetric work than ever before. Doctor Hugh, himself, was appointed in the year of publication to the post of Physician-in-Ordinary to the King. (To Charles II, that is, who was extraordinarily productive of babies.) Inevitably, the Chamberlens' renewed success aroused afresh the fierce hostility of the officials of the College of Physicians, most of whom would have given their right ears for the royal job in which Doctor Hugh had got himself so comfortably ensconced.

For fifteen years, the angry physicians had to wait for their chance to get their own back on Doctor Hugh. Then, in 1688, he was asked to appear before the Comitia of the College and was accused of practising medicine without a proper licence. Oh, but he had been appointed Physician-in-Ordinary to the King, had he not? was his rejoinder. Was not the royal seal a sufficient authority? Mr Chamberlen's appointment had been to the *last* king, retorted the officials of the College. Now that there was a new king, they declared, he had no standing as a physician at all.

Having established that, to their own satisfaction, they asked him to account for the death of a Mrs Phoebe Willmer, of Friday Street, London—a woman, normally, of 'a very healthy and cheerful constitution'. Mr Willmer, called to give evidence, deposed that his wife

... Being taken ill of a paine in her right side under her short ribb together with a great difficulty of breathing having but 14 weeks to go with Child Mr Hugh Chamberlen Senr was sent for to take care of her, who thereupon gave her in the space of nine days four vomitts, four purges, and caused her to be bled three times to the quantity of eight ounces each time: Then gave her something to raise a spitting after which swellings and Ulcers in her mouth followed; about 3 or 4 days after her taking this, she miscarried, and it was attended with a looseness and she continued languishing till she dyed. Soon after she was brought to bed the Nails of her fingers grew crooked, the skin from her feet and fingers all scaled off. The Patient's Husband proposed to him [ie to Hugh Chamberlen Senior] to have the advice of a Physician, but he refused it, Speaking very much in his own praise saying that no Physician could do the Cures [which] he had done & very much villefied other Physicians . . .

Although he tried to defend himself, Hugh Chamberlen was found Guilty of Mal Praxis, fined 'Ten Pounds of lawfull money of England', and ordered to stay in Newgate Gaol until the money was paid. (Chamberlen promptly put his hand in his pocket and pulled out sufficient gold.) This does not seem to have affected in any way the faith that members of the Royal Family had in his abilities—he was asked to be present at the birth of the child who was to become the Old Pretender, but arrived an hour too late; in 1692 he attended the confinement of Princess Anne of Denmark, receiving a fee of one hundred guineas in spite of the fact that the child died immediately after the birth. Meanwhile, in France, Julien Clement had attended Mme de Montespan at the birth of the Duc de Maine in 1670, and had delivered the Dauphine in 1682. There is no doubt that the example set by these prominent ladies led to the gradual acceptance of the man-midwife, during the eighteenth century, by those who were considerably less exalted.

The process may have been hastened, rather than delayed, by Hugh Chamberlen's preoccupation with an extraordinary scheme that had nothing to do with obstetrics at all. His proposal—'To make England Rich and Happy'—was published in 1690 and, after that, absorbed his entire attention for nearly ten years. (He was 'pre-eminently conspicuous among the political mountebanks, whose busy faces were seen every day in the lobby of the House of Commons', according to Lord Macaulay.) Chamberlen wanted a Land Bank:

> . . . A Land Bank would work for England miracles such as had never been wrought for Israel, miracles exceeding the heaps of quails and the daily shower of manna. There would be no taxes, and yet the exchequer would be full to overflowing. There would be no poor rates: for there would be no poor. The income of every landowner would be doubled. The profits of every merchant would be increased. In short, the island would . . . be the paradise of the world . . . These blessed effects the Land Bank was to produce simply by issuing

enormous quantities of notes on landed security. The doctrine of the projectors was that every person who had real property ought to have, beside that property, paper money to the full value of that property. Thus, if his estate was worth two thousand pounds, he ought to have his estate and two thousand pounds in paper money . . .

In 1699 it was rumoured in London that Doctor Chamberlen, 'the manmidwife and sole contriver and manager of the Land Bank, is retired to Holland, on suspition of debt'. Lampoons were published, accusing him of making off with the funds of the bank. It is not certain that Hugh Chamberlen did actually cross the Channel as soon as he disappeared from the London scene, for he is known to have been pressing his Land Bank project on the Scottish parliament in 1700, and two years after that he was urging the union of Scotland with England—ironically, the only one of the Chamberlens' grandiose plans that actually came to fruition.

Eventually, however, Hugh Chamberlen did reach Holland, and there, to a man named Rogier van Roonhuysen, he parted with the precious family secret—probably, in exchange for enough money to remove the 'suspition of debt'.* Van Roonhuysen used the forceps profitably himself for a number of years, but he was unable or unwilling to guard the secret as carefully as the senior members of the Chamberlen family had done for nearly a century. By 1733, when the first illustrated account of the use of the forceps was published, a large number of practitioners in various parts of north-west Europe were skilled in the use of the implement. These practitioners were professionally qualified and invariably male, and, in spite of the traditional barriers that had been erected for so long against the presence of men at childbirth, were in great demand in the lying-in room. The scientific study of pregnancy and parturition could, thanks to the failure of the Land Bank scheme, all too belatedly begin.

Woodham Mortimer Hall, once the home of Doctor Peter Chamberlen ('The Third'), continued to be the property of some member of the Chamberlen family until about the year 1715, when it was sold by one Hope Chamberlen to a Mr William Alexander,

* This is the story as given by early medical historians. Modern scholars have suggested that van Roonhuysen may have learned the Chamberlens' secret before this.

a wine merchant. When he died, Mr Alexander bequeathed the estate to the Wine Coopers' Company.

In 1813 a Mrs Kemball happened to visit her daughter, who was living at that time at the Hall. Quite by chance, Mrs Kemball went into an unused closet above the entrance porch. Looking round, she noticed, and had her interest taken by, a small cork or wooden disc that appeared to have been let into the floor. Near it, she saw a second cork or disc, which was apparently in line with the first. When the two circular inlays were investigated and removed, it was found that each had been used to cover and conceal a large screw-head. When the enquiry was continued, a trapdoor with small sunken hinges was revealed. When the trapdoor was raised, the researchers found beneath it a cavity, formed between the floor and the ceiling timbers beneath. In the cavity, carefully hidden, they found several coins; a medallion of King Charles I or II; a miniature painting of Doctor Peter Chamberlen that had been much damaged by time; a tooth wrapped in paper on which was written 'My Husband's Last Tooth'; a little antique plate; a pair of lady's long yellow kid gloves, in an excellent state of preservation; and ... some boxes in which were (with some other quite primitive instruments) three pairs of midwifery forceps. Without any doubt at all, these were the forceps used so secretly and so profitably by the one-time owner of the Hall and by his father and his uncle.

Long before 1813, the midwives, so long entrenched in their exclusive monopoly, had started to fight back against the physicians' attempts to interfere with what the good women regarded as their 'rights'. Wherever a 'man-midwife', a 'mid-man', a 'surgeon man-midwife' or an 'andro-boethogynist' started to attract customers, he could be sure to meet with ridicule, or worse, from the members of the sisterhood most nearly affected. A Mrs Sarah Stone, a Mrs Kennon and a Mrs Elizabeth Blackwell are said to have been particularly belligerent.

The midwives must have been amused, rather than alarmed, by a book written by John Maubray, and published in 1724. Maubray, who was probably the first teacher of practical midwifery in Britain, and who was certainly the first medical man to suggest the building of a special lying-in hospital in his native land, called his book *The Female Physician, containing all the diseases incident to that*

Sex, in virgins, wives and widows; together with their causes and symptoms, their Degrees of Danger, and respective methods of Prevention and Cure: to which is added, The whole Art of New Improved Midwifery; comprehending the necessary qualifications of a Midwife, and particular directions for lying-in women, in all cases of Difficult and Preternatural Births; together with the Diet and Regimen of both the Mother and Child.

Maubray's system of midwifery may have been 'new' and 'improved', but his book contained certain demonstrable fallacies. In the chapter on 'Deformed Conceptions and Monsters, Etc'— abnormalities caused, Maubray said, by indecent conjugal relations—the author gave an account of a remarkable little beast called a 'Sucker' which he had seen issue from the womb of a woman he had attended when she had been in labour on a 'fare-vessel' on the Zuider Zee. The monster had been 'the likeliest of anything in shape and size to a Moodiwarp, having a hooked snout, fiery sparkling eyes, a long round neck, an acuminated short tail and an extraordinary agility of feet'. At its first sight of the world's light a Sucker would yell and shriek fearfully, added Maubray. Then, seeking a lurking hole, it would run up and down like a little demon, 'which indeed I took it for the first time I saw it, and *that* none of the better sort.' The author had been informed by 'some of the most learned men' that this 'little yelling demon' was so common among the seafaring and meaner sort of people that scarce one mother in three escaped its extraordinary visitation.

A more extraordinary visitation even than that brought fame (or notoriety) to a woman named Mary Tofts, who was a native of Godalming, near Guildford, in the County of Surrey.

Mrs Tofts was the wife of a journeyman clothier. She first showed signs of abnormality on 23 April 1726, when:

... As she was weeding in a Field, she saw a Rabbet [rabbit] spring up near her after which she ran with another Woman that was at work just by her: this set her a longing for Rabbets, being then, as she thought, five Weeks gone with Child; the other Woman perceiving she was uneasy, charged her with longing for the Rabbet they cou'd not catch, but she deny'd it: soon after another Rabbet sprung up near the same place, which she endeavour'd likewise to catch. The same Night she dreamt that she was in a Field with those two Rabbets in her

Lap and awaked with a sick Fit which lasted till Morning; from that time for above three Months, she had a constant and strong desire to eat Rabbits, but being very poor and indigent cou'd not procure any . . .

Mrs Tofts' springtime uneasiness seemed to have been quite justified when, during the following November, she took to her bed and, in due time, was delivered of a litter of seventeen rabbits. She was attended, during her very unusual confinement, by John Howard, the local apothecary, who had been practising midwifery for the past thirty years without seeing any woman give birth to rabbits before. Not doubting for one single moment that this miraculous parturition, though unprecedented in his experience, was entirely genuine, Howard sent a description of the case to his friend, Nathaniel St André, who was practising at that time at the newly established Westminster Hospital.

St André was a native of Switzerland who had been brought to England in the entourage of a wealthy Jewish family. After trying several different methods of earning a living—he was, for a short time, a professional dancing master—he had set himself up, though not properly qualified, as a medical man and, because of his knowledge of the German language, had been appointed by King George I 'Anatomist to the Royal Household'.

As quickly as he could after he received the momentous news of Mrs Tofts' delivery, St André left for Godalming, taking with him another friend, Samuel Molyneux, who happened to be Secretary to the Prince of Wales. The two London men looked wonderingly at Mrs Tofts. They looked wonderingly at the remains of her prodigious family. They talked earnestly and at length to the apothecary Howard:

> . . . Mr Howard further related that when she [Mrs Tofts] was delivered of one Rabbet, another was immediately felt in her Belly struggling with such Violence, that the Motion thereof cou'd be sensibly felt and seen . . .

Then St André, seeing in the case (as we might say nowadays) a quick buck or two for himself, wrote and rushed off to the printer's an authoritative pamphlet, which he entitled *A Short*

Narrative of an Extraordinary Delivery of Rabbets . . . published by Mr St André, Surgeon and Anatomist to His Majesty, London, 1727, 8vo.

In this pamphlet, which was well larded with rather pretentious medical jargon, St André described how he himself had delivered the woman of two rabbits, or portions thereof, and he appended to it a note promising that 'The Account of the Delivery of the Eighteenth Rabbet shall be published by way of Appendix to this Account'.

As soon as the pamphlet appeared and was offered for sale in the streets of London, news of Mrs Tofts' phenomenal achievement spread round the capital like wildfire. Some citizens were impressed, others were sceptical. 'I want to know what faith you have in the miracle at Guildford,' wrote Alexander Pope to a friend. 'All London is divided into factions about it.' Many courtiers believed St André's story to be true. Others, following the example of the Prince of Wales, sniggered quietly behind their hands.

Among the doubters was the monarch himself—George 1— Teutonic and matter-of-fact. He, not wholly convinced by his Surgeon and Anatomist's pamphlet, sent another of his personal medical men—one Cyriacus Ahlers—into Surrey to investigate the matter. Ahlers examined the productive lady so thoroughly that he was able to remove from the approaches to her womb a portion of yet another rabbit. The local apothecary, possibly resenting these repeated incursions into his personal territory, accused the London man of treating his patient boorishly. Ahlers, taking offence, immediately returned to London, where he gave a non-committal account to the king.

As the matter—from the point of view of the capital—was still undecided, the king, who had a Germanic urge to know everything *for certain*, and was vigorously egged on by his wife, then sent into Surrey Sir Richard Manningham, who was one of the most noted physician-accoucheurs of the day.

Manningham, who had been ordered by the king to report fully and impartially on the case, decided at once that Mrs Tofts was an impostor. Probably, Manningham guessed, the woman had artfully concealed the fifteen famous rabbit-children around her person before she had ostensibly given birth to them. He did not say this, though. On the contrary, he flattered Mrs Tofts. He offered to take her up to London, where she would be seen by (among others) the king . . .

All unsuspecting, the Godalming celebrity swallowed Manningham's bait. On 29 November 1726—less than a month after she had so suddenly become so famous—she travelled to the metropolis under the auspices of the royal doctor and was lodged by him there in Lacy's 'Bagnio' (or, as we would probably say nowadays, 'nursing home') in Leicester Fields—better known, now, as Leicester Square.

During the next three days and three nights, every move made by Mrs Tofts was watched closely from every possible viewing point. On her fourth day in London, Mrs Tofts made a fatal mistake. She sent a messenger out from the Bagnio with secret instructions that her errand-runner should go to the market in Covent Garden and should procure for her, there, a *rabbit*.

At once, there was an uproar. Examined and severely threatened by Sir Thomas Clarges, a Justice of the Peace, in the presence of Manningham, the Duke of Montague, Doctor James Douglas, and other witnesses, Mrs Tofts made a full confession of her duplicity. Then, she was committed for a short while to the Bridewell lock-up in Tothill Fields and was told that she would be prosecuted under a Statute of Edward III as a vile cheat and impostor. The trial was not proceeded with, however, and soon she was allowed to go back, considerably chastened, to Godalming.

Shortly after Mrs Tofts had returned home in disgrace from the big city, Manningham published a pamphlet entitled *An Exact Diary of what was observed during a close attendance upon Mary Toft the pretended Rabbit Breeder*. In this work, Manningham managed to demonstrate that the pieces of rabbit produced as evidence in the case were fragments of adult coney, not of newly-born beast. He did not tell his readers, though, whether Mrs Tofts was a dishonest rogue, or just a poor hysterical subject attempting to attract notice to herself by extraordinary means. Conceivably, he did not know.

Manningham came quite well out of the business, attracting so much attention to himself by his *Exact Diary* that he was soon able to pick and choose between potential patients. He was particularly unwilling to travel far out of town in his professional affairs.

(Laurence Sterne, in *The Life and Opinions of Tristram Shandy, Gentleman*, described him as 'the famous Dr Manningham' who, as Mrs Shandy was determined to lie-in in the country, 'was not to be had'.) St André, on the other hand, lost so much face that he only once ventured to present himself at Court after the scandal, and though he retained the position of 'Anatomist to the King' he never again drew the salary attached to the post. Within three years, he had been forced to withdraw to an obscure retreat in the country.

William Smellie, who was (we can see now) a key figure in the history of obstetrics, was not quite so obvious a butt for the midwives' fun as John Maubray or Nathaniel St André, but he managed to rouse the particularly virulent scorn of Mrs Elizabeth Nihell, who practised her trade round London's Hay Market. Mrs Nihell referred publicly to Smellie as 'a great horse-godmother of a he-midwife' and tried to make him look ridiculous by describing him 'with his figure softened by his pocket nightgown of flowered calico or his cap of office tied with silk and silver ribbon'. Her taunts were a tribute to the remarkable man's efficiency and capacity for work.

Smellie was born at Lanark, in Scotland, and he may have studied at Glasgow. (He is known to have graduated there as Doctor of Medicine on 18 February 1745.) For a short time he busied himself with a general practice in Lanark and the country around, carrying in his pocket tincture of castor, spirits of hartshorn and liquid laudanum in separate bottles and compounding his medicine on the spot from one, two or three of these ingredients. He did not hesitate to practise operative surgery when this was needed. (A bill of his still exists, for 'seven pound sterling for amputation and cure of your leg; make thankfull payt. and oblige your humble servt., Wil. Smellie'.)

In 1738—feeling, perhaps, that Lanark and the surrounding country did not afford sufficient scope for his undoubted talents—Smellie left Scotland by the 'finest road' and travelled to London. A year later, he went to Paris and attended a course of lectures given by the well-known French obstetrician Jean Grégoire. When he returned to London, he started to practise in Pall Mall in premises that one of his most prejudiced critics called 'a very mean apothecary's shop'.

As well as being a highly accomplished man-midwife, Smellie was an inspiring teacher. He had no influential friends in London when he arrived there, and no connection with any hospital, clinic or dispensing-rooms. He simply attended poor pregnant women, in their own homes, and he took his students with him. (In a ten-year period, he is believed to have had more than nine hundred pupils, instructing them in over eleven hundred cases of labour.) The critic referred to above says that Smellie had a paper lantern hanging outside his house with 'Midwifery Taught For Five Shillings' written on it. That critic, as we have said, was prejudiced, but he was probably, in this respect at least, quite accurate. Only rarely, in all the fields of human endeavour, can so much have been taught for so negligible a sum.

In the researches he made into the varying predicaments of his eleven hundred poor lying-in women, Smellie was able to establish—more exactly, perhaps, than anyone had ever been able to do before—what actually happened to the baby or babies during parturition. He was able to do this because he was able to study more closely than any male had previously been allowed to the curves followed by the infant in the last stages of a woman's pregnancy and during its birth.

In order to be able to explain the more clearly to his students what was happening in each delivery, Smellie constructed a dummy or 'machine' made of real human bones covered with leather, through which an articulated 'manikin' or artificial foetus could be propelled on its simulated journey. (Sir Richard Manningham had had a similar teaching-aid. Probably, that gave Smellie the idea.) Realizing that he would probably want to publish the results of his researches, Smellie made copious and exact notes of every unusual case he and his students encountered. His classic *Treatise on the Theory and Practice of Midwifery*, prepared from these notes and published in 1752, appeared in at least nine English editions and was translated into French, German and Dutch.

Difficult births, Smellie taught, could be due to one of two frequently-encountered causes. Possibly, he said—and he was able to demonstrate this on his 'machine'—the child was being presented ready for delivery in an impossibly difficult position. Normally, he showed, the top of the child's head would appear first, and this would make mechanically for the easiest delivery. Labour would be longer and more painful if the child lay backwards in the womb. In a certain percentage of the cases he attended with his students, the baby's face might appear first, instead of the top of its head—or, worse, its buttocks (a 'breech presentation'). In some really bad presentations—they occurred approximately once in every two hundred and fifty births—the child would lie transversely across the passage, and if its position were not changed the birth would be completely prevented. When that had happened in less enlightened times than the middle of the eighteenth century, taught Smellie, the midwives concerned would have tried desperately to turn the child. Hopelessly drunk (probably), and without any real knowledge of what was happening, they would have suspended the unfortunate mother-to-be by her arms, and they would have violently kneaded her abdomen. Their efforts would have been only rarely successful, and most pregnant women who were caught in this ghastly predicament and were unable to escape from it would have died in the most terrible agony.

By 1751 there was not quite so much danger of this happening. Obstetrical techniques had not altered much since Herodotus recorded the methods of the Ancient Egyptians, but 'podalic version', at least, was part of any normally-skilled midwife's stock-in-trade. In this operation, the midwife would put a hand, somehow, into the mother's womb and would draw the feet of the awkwardly-placed infant down, first, out of the uterus mouth. It was not an easy operation to perform and, in fact, the sheer physical strength required may have helped to turn public opinion in favour of the male accoucheur. (François Mauriceau, man-midwife to French queens, said that the difficulties of this kind of labour often made him sweat in the middle of winter.)

Podalic version carried out by an unskilled midwife could be hazardous. William Lowder, who towards the end of the eighteenth century used to lecture on midwifery in St Saviour's Churchyard, Southwark, was fond of quoting one instance of strength wrongly used by a midwife who, in turning a child, pulled too violently on one foot. Being unable to deliver the baby, she sent for a gentleman, who managed to turn the child and to bring it away:

... The good midwife offered the child to the gentleman and said 'Oh, Sir, look here!', when he saw that one of the child's feet was off, at which he was very much astonished. Now the midwife it was that had pulled the child's foot off before she had sent for the gentleman and had put it in her pocket! ...

Podalic version was much easier to do when it could be tried out on Mr Smellie's life-size model first.

Mr Smellie was not very keen on the use of the 'cranioclast'—an instrument that had been developed for those awful occasions when a baby's head presented, but was too large to pass through the opening in the mother's pelvis, or when the pelvic opening of the mother was so abnormally narrow that it afforded no proper passage for the unborn infant's skull, even if this were of quite normal dimensions. Delivery with the cranioclast was a sickening and messy business—with this horrible tool, the skull of the unborn baby would be broken open, which would kill the infant, after which the contents of the skull would be extracted. The skull-bones would be forced together, next, so that the body of the dead baby could be removed fairly easily from the womb. Mr Smellie objected to this ingenious instrument principally because it was all too liable to damage the internal tissues of the lady into which it was being inserted.

Mr Smellie approved of the Chamberlens' midwifery forceps, though—so much so, that he devised a novel pair of boxwood forceps of his own in which the blades locked together without the use of a screw or any kind of mechanical pivot. ('The English Lock', this was afterwards called.) Shortly after that, he produced two pairs of leather-covered iron forceps—a short version, which was curved in one direction only, to suit the shape of the head of the child, and a pair with longer blades which were intended to follow the curve of the mother's pelvis. Soon, most of Mr Smellie's pupils were busy designing obstetric forceps to conform to their own ideas of what was wanted. By 1760 there were nearly as many different types of forceps in use (it was unkindly claimed) as there were man-midwives.

Laurence Sterne, the clergyman-author of *Tristram Shandy*, seized with delight on the new craze. Doctor Slop, the man-midwife who carried his beloved instruments in a 'green bays bag' and used them even when they were not necessary, is one of the most amusing characters in that hilariously funny book. (He was drawn 'from life', Sterne's model being a Doctor Burton, a well-known practitioner with Jacobite sympathies.) Sterne enjoyed depicting the father of the unborn Tristram, too—Mr Shandy, retired Turkey Merchant, who, dipping into some quasi-learned tome, had discovered that:

> ... The lax and pliable state of a child's head in parturition, the bones of the cranium having no sutures at that time, was such, —that by force of the woman's efforts, which, in strong labour-pains, was equal, upon an average, to the weight of 470 pounds avoirdupois acting perpendicularly upon it;—it so happened, that in 49 instances out of 50, the said head was compressed and moulded into the shape of an oblong conical piece of dough, such as a pastry-cook generally rolls up in order to make a pye of ...

Having learned that such terrible dangers faced his son, Mr Shandy studied further and read of the operation by which Julius Caesar, Scipio Africanus, Manlius Torquatus, King Edward VI and others had, allegedly, come sideways into the world. The incision of the *abdomen* and *uterus* ran 'for six weeks together' in Mr Shandy's head, until he was satisfied that:

> ... Wounds in the *epigastrium*, and those in the *matrix*, were not mortal;—so that the belly of the mother might be opened extremely well to give a passage to the child ...

Rashly, he mentioned the matter one afternoon to Mrs Shandy, merely as a matter of fact:

> ... But seeing her turn as pale as ashes at the very mention of it, as much as the operation flattered his hopes,—he thought it as well to say no more of it,—contenting himself with admiring, —what he thought was to no purpose to propose ...

In real life—as opposed to Laurence Sterne's fun-world—there was very little to be said for delivery 'by Caesarean section' in the hopelessly septic conditions of the dirty, unaired and over-heated eighteenth-century lying-in room. Being *always* fatal to the mother, said Sir Richard Manningham, the operation should only be performed after her death, to save the child, if it were possible for the child to be saved.

William Osborne, Doctor of Medicine and man-midwife to the Lying-In Hospital in Store Street, London, said that no one could possibly justify the use of a Caesarean operation. If the mother's pelvis measured less than three inches 'in the conjugate diameter', he said, the head of the unborn child should be reduced in size by craniotomy in the usual way, after which the lifeless carcase should be removed from the womb with a crotchet, or with forceps. In exceptionally difficult cases, the baby's body could be left to putrefy in the uterus, so that it would become soft and, therefore, could be the more easily delivered. To support his thesis, Osborne quoted a case of extreme contraction of the pelvis where the distance between the symphisis and the base of the sacrum was only three quarters of an inch. The patient was in labour for three days, he said, and was repeatedly examined by several doctors and by over thirty students. After its head had been shrunk, the child's body was left in the good woman's uterus for thirty-six hours before it was delivered 'by the crochet', the operation lasting for about three hours. The patient acknowledged on the seventh day that she was then 'as well as in any period of her life'. Osborne, of course, was delighted. This and two similar cases proved (he concluded) 'that it is possible to deliver a child, when the head is lessened, through almost any pelvis, however small its dimensions may be; and therefore that the Caesarean section can hardly become necessary simply on account of the capacity of the pelvis'.

Sir Fielding Ould (1710–89), Master of the Lying-In Hospital in Dublin, declared that the Caesarean section was a 'detestable, barbarous, illegal piece of inhumanity', though he was realistic enough to admit that in extreme cases of pelvic contraction both mother and child would perish if the detestable and barbarous operation were not performed. 'Whether we should destroy the mother to save the child is a deplorable dilemma which should certainly be cleared up by the divines,' wrote Ould, surely aware that the Doctors of Theology of the University of Paris had published an evasive report on the subject, from the Sorbonne, as far back as 1733. The Caesarean operation was performed successfully only once in the British Isles before 1793 (when a Doctor Barlow, of Bolton, carried it off, though losing the child). The earlier, almost miraculous instance was in January 1739, when Mary Donally, an ignorant country midwife, managed to save both the mother under her care and protection, and the baby. Doubtless, as this happened in Ireland, a saint or some other supernatural being was coping with the hitherto unsolved problem of sepsis.

Puerperal fever—a general blood-poisoning that originates from childbirth or miscarriage—has been known under various names since (at least) the days of Hippocrates. In 1651 William Harvey, the distinguished London physician who first established the fact that the blood circulates, described the puerperal sickness in sickening terms:

> ... For it often befalls a woman [he said] especially the more tender sort, that the after-purgings being corrupted and grown noisome do call in Feavers and other grievous symptoms ... If any part of the after-burden be left sticking to the uterus the after-purgings will flow forth evil-sented, green and as if they proceeded from a dead body: and sometimes the courage and strength of the womb being quite vanquished, a suddaine Gangrene doth induce a certain death ...

Harvey had some success in the case of 'a very honourable lady' who had the fever when he tried 'immitting an injection' into her with a little syringe 'whereupon black clotted and noisome blood did issue out even to some certain pounds weight, whereby she received present ease'.

In spite of this happy outcome, puerperal fever was still inducing certain deaths, and all too many of them throughout the eighteenth century. The mortality figures that have come down to us from the few maternity hospitals that existed at the time are quite shocking: out of the sixty-five women delivered at the New Westminster Lying-In Hospital in London during the period between 30 November 1769 and 15 May 1770, for instance, nineteen were affected by the 'childbed fever', and fourteen died.

John Leake, who had helped to found the hospital and was its first physician, broke new ground by suggesting that the beds in his and other hospitals should not be too numerous, that the wards should be well ventilated, and that the patients should be supplied with clean linen. In spite of his recommendations, the fever continued to claim its victims.

A lot of the credit for conquering the perils of puerperal infection must go to Charles White, whose description of a typical eighteenth-century lying-in room was given at the beginning of this chapter.

White was born in Manchester in 1728. After studying for some time with his father, who had been appointed doctor to the poor of Manchester and the surrounding districts and was particularly interested in midwifery, White Junior went to London to attend the lectures on anatomy given by Doctor William Hunter. After a further period of study in Edinburgh, where a small school of obstetrics was being formed, White Junior returned to his native city to join his father in practice.

According to Thomas De Quincey, one of the younger White's patients died when he was twenty-nine years of age, leaving him, by her will, £25,000 on condition that her body was to be embalmed and kept above ground for one hundred years, and that once a year White, with two witnesses present, should withdraw the veil from her face. The lady was accordingly mummified and placed in a clock-case in White's anatomical museum. From there, she was moved, later, to an attic in the large mansion called The Priory, at Sale, that he purchased with part of his bequest. (After several further changes of resting-place, the lady's body was finally interred in 1868 in the Cemetery at Harpurhey, on the outskirts of Manchester.)

White survived his benefactress by fifty-six years. During nearly the whole of that time, he went on enlarging the practice he had taken over from his father, modestly attributing his success to the splendid example his father had set him, and to the correctness of the methods his father had taught. But the younger White's pioneering work was entirely his own:

> ... In hospitals [he said] if separate apartments cannot be allowed to every patient, at least as soon as the fever has seized

one, she ought immediately to be removed into another room, not only for her immediate safety, but for that of the other patients; or, it would be better still if every woman were delivered in a separate ward and was to remain there a week or ten days until all danger of this fever is over . . .

By 1773 White was arguably the greatest obstetrician in the world. In that year, when he made public the results of his researches in his authoritative *Treatise on the Management of Pregnant and Lying-in Women, and the means of Curing, but more especially of Preventing the Principle Disorders of which they are Liable*, he was able to claim that in his extensive experience of more than twenty years, while cases of puerperal fever had occurred through non-observance of the rules he had laid down, he had never lost a patient from this disease. White's book—which, says the *Dictionary of National Biography*, effected a revolution in the practice of midwifery, rescuing it from semi-barbarism and placing it on a rational and humane basis—went through four editions in England within twenty years, was translated into French and German, and was reprinted in America in 1793.

Just before the end of the century, a Doctor Alexander Gordon published a *Treatise on the Epidemic Puerperal Fever of Aberdeen*. Gordon knew that women were free from the disease until *after* delivery. In his book, he advanced the theory that:

. . . Till that time there is no inlet open to receive the infectious matter which produces the disease; but after delivery the matter is readily and copiously admitted by the numerous patulous [wide] orifices which are open to imbibe it, by the separation of the placenta from the uterus . . .

William Harvey, squirting away busily with his 'little syringe' into his 'very honourable lady' back in 1651 had suggested long before Alexander Gordon, that the uterus might be the seat of the trouble. William Smellie had agreed, more or less (or it might be due to 'obstruction of the lochia', he said). The great William Hunter, in his turn, had decided that the disease was a form of peritonitis. Gordon waved aside Hunter's theories and guided all subsequent research firmly back into the path indicated by

William Harvey. Gordon had noticed, too, that there seemed to be some kind of connection between puerperal fever and erysipelas. Alexander Hamilton, Professor of Midwifery at Edinburgh from 1780 to 1800 was also aware of the erysipelas-puerperal fever link:

> ... It is particularly observed in surgical wards [he wrote] that there is such a state of the air sometimes as produces almost in every wound, even the slightest, symptoms of erysipelas and even mortification. In the Edinburgh Infirmary, when the lying-in ward was there, it was observed that when such a state of the air was present, puerperal fever raged violently, but at no other time ...

Gordon earned a small but honourable niche in medical history by emphatically recommending the disinfection of the lying-in chamber. 'The nurses and the physicians who have attended patients affected with the puerperal fever ought carefully to wash themselves and to get their apparel properly fumigated before it be put on again,' he instructed. It was 1850 before Sir James Simpson was to publish his classical essay on the subject, but men like Leake, White, Hamilton and Gordon had effectively pointed the way.

4

The Nursery Jungle

. . . The hand that rocks the cradle
Is the hand that rules the world . . .

WILLIAM ROSS WALLACE, d. 1881

It is difficult for us today, with our problems of over-population, to appreciate fully the appallingly high death rate among children in the eighteenth century. Thomas Gibbon the historian computed —rather imprecisely, for an historian—that 'the greater part are snatched away before their ninth year'. (He himself lost five brothers and a sister who all died in infancy.) Two-thirds of the children born in the Metropolitan Area of London in the eighteenth century died before they were five years old—we know that, now, from figures printed in the *Gentleman's Magazine*—and three out of every four of these poor little victims failed to reach even their second birthdays. In the eighth edition of William Buchan's *Domestic Medicine*, published as late in the century as 1784, we can see these ominous words:

> . . . It appears from the annual register of the dead that almost one half of the children born in Great Britain die under twelve years of age . . .

As we have seen, to survive the perils of parturition during the eighteenth century, an infant had to be extraordinarily lucky or extraordinarily tough—and, usually, it had to be both. To survive its first few hours of life it needed a much more resilient digestive system than any new-born baby would require today.

For it would not be allowed to lie quietly in its cot or cradle until it had had a chance to recover from the exhausting adventure it had just undergone, and until its mother was ready and willing to feed it from her own natural sources of nourishment. As soon as it was born, the eighteenth-century baby was thought to be hungry, and it would be given, or forcibly fed with, some horrible concoction known in England and America as 'pap'. (Bread or flour soaked in milk, or in water, or in both, usually formed the basis of pap. Sometimes, beer was an ingredient. Occasionally, the pap would be pre-chewed by the nurse.) Alternatively, the baby might be given a 'posset' made of flour and sugar, or oil of sweet almonds, or syrup of violets. In some cases it might have to survive, within its first hour or two of life, the administration of a liberal 'comforter' compounded of butter and sugar, or of some 'cordial' or 'caudle' (usually, the alcoholic mess with which the midwife and her assistants had been sustaining themselves.)

Once it had recovered from the shock of its birth and from the after-effects of its first meals, the eighteenth-century infant had to be prepared, dietetically speaking, for practically anything. When it was offered milk—which seems to us, today, so obviously suitable as a source of nourishment for the very young—the precious fluid might well have been tested first for its suitability by a rudimentary method described nearly two thousand years ago in the writings of Soranus of Ephesus, and repeated by Thomas Phaer in 1545 in the first book on the diseases of children to be written in English:

> . . . That mylke is goode that is whyte and sweete; and when ye droppe it on your nayle and do move your finger, neyther fleteth abrod at every stiring nor will hang faste, upon your naile, when ye turne it downeward, but that whyche is betwene is beste . . .

William Smellie ('The great horse godmother of a man-midwife') was recommending the use of this simple test even as late as 1752.

How lucky was the eighteenth-century infant that was fed regularly on good milk that was 'whyte and sweete', and on that alone! There was an odds-on chance that it would have to put up with pap and yet more pap, until it was ready to be weaned on to 'solid' foods. Richard Conyers, physician to Captain Thomas Coram's Foundling Hospital in London and one of the first men anywhere to recognize that the traditional methods of feeding might be wrong, said in 1748 that pap was a mess which might be much more usefully employed by bookbinders in sticking pages together than given to infants as nourishment.

As a palliative, there was an odds-on chance that the pap-fed infant would be given Daffy's *Elexir*, Godfrey's *Cordial*, Dalby's *Carminative*, or some other proprietary soother.

Daffy's *Elexir* was a stock remedy for all infant ills. It is said to have been originated by the Reverend Thomas Daffy, one-time Rector of Redmile in the Vale of Belvoir. The good clergyman's daughter carried on its manufacture after her father's death, advertising:

> ... The true Elexir is sold at the *Hand and Pen* in Maiden-lane, Covent Garden and at many Coffee-houses, also at Mr John Waters, Perfumer at the *Naked Boy and Orange Tree*, near the Maypole in the Strand ...

There were several rival makers of the infants' cure-all, among them being one John Harrison of Prujean's Court in London's Old Bailey, who, in 1709, charged Mrs Elizabeth Daffy with making 'invidious remarks upon his *Elexir Salutis*'. Mrs Daffy issued counter-charges, claiming that Harrison had pretended falsely to have been her late husband's assistant in the preparation of the elixir. According to the wrappers round the bottles in which it was sold, the genuine remedy was 'much recommended to the public by Dr King, physician to King Charles ii, and the late learned and ingenious Dr Radcliffe'. It was compounded of senna, jalap, aniseed, caraway seeds and juniper berries steeped in alcohol, to which treacle and water were added. It was widely sold and used in America.

Godfrey's *Cordial*, also very popular in America, was probably as lethal as any of the noisome concoctions with which the eighteenth-century infant might be dosed, solely to keep the house quiet. The word 'cordial' was itself dangerously misleading —how, asked one Censor of the College of Physicians in London, could anyone suspect any mischief from a medicine with so harm-less-sounding a name? But, Godfrey's attractive mixture relied principally for its effectiveness on opium. And opium, as Doctor A Hume pointed out in his book *Every Woman her Own Physician*, published in 1776, was not really a suitable substance to find in a nursery medicine chest:

> ... Nearly all the children who die within the first year are carried off by convulsions but then these convulsions are the consequence of other disorders which justly demand the utmost attention and care of the mother or nurse who are entrusted with so precious a charge as the life and health of the little innocents. Humanity obliges the author to speak plainly upon this subject and he is sure he shall not offend the worthy and the good by declaring that those convulsions which carry off thousands of infants every year are chiefly owing to the brutality and laziness of nurses who are for ever pouring *Godfrey's Cordial* down their little throats, which is a strong opiate and in the end as fatal as Arsenic. This they will pretend they do to quiet the child—*thus indeed many are for ever quieted*—when the negligent parents (who put their children out to nurse because they would not be disturbed with their affecting cries) are acquainted that the little babe went off suddenly in convulsions, and all parties are perfectly satisfied. If such a conduct is not *murder* I know not what is ...

Few people seem to have realized, before the end of the eighteenth century, that the vessels from which babies were fed ought to be clean, and that glass was, therefore, a specially suitable material for making them. Until the need for more hygienic conditions was appreciated, babies not fed from the breast had to take into their tiny and very vulnerable mouths teat-substitutes made of horn, wood, pewter or some other germ-laden material. George Armstrong, who opened in 1769 the first institution for sick children in Britain—a 'Dispensary for the Infant Poor' at a house in London's Red Lion Square—examined the problem of infant-feeding in some detail without managing to suggest a method that might keep more of the poor little dears alive:

> ... There are two ways of feeding children who are bred up by the hand: the one is by means of a horn, and the other is with a boat or spoon. They both have their advocates, but the latter in my humble opinion is preferable.
> The horn made use of for sucking is a small polished cow's

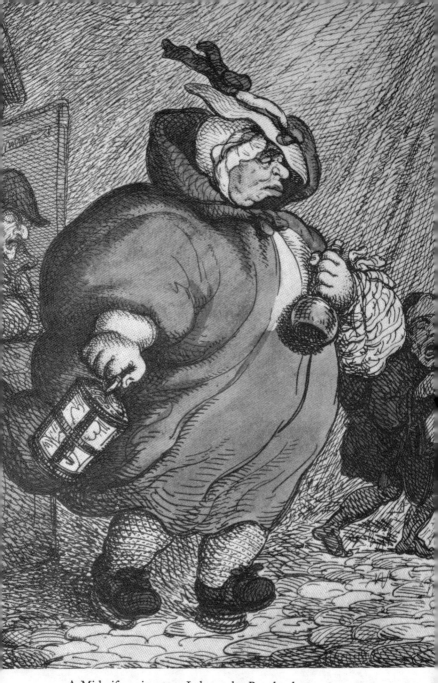

A Midwife going to a Labour, by Rowlandson, 1811.

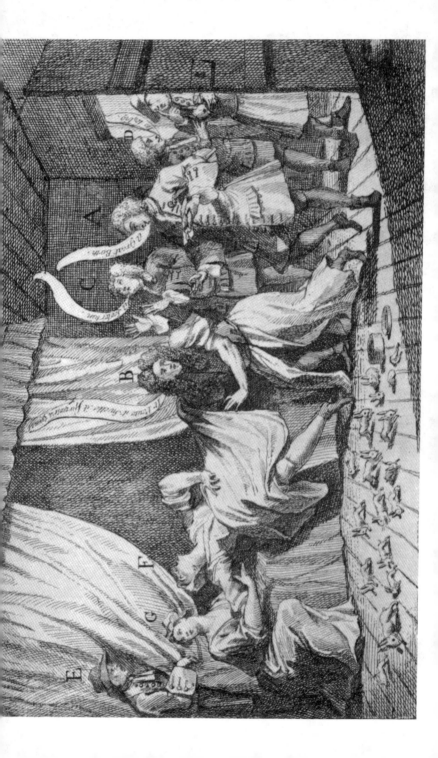

horn which will hold about a gill and a half. The small end of it is perforated and has a notch round it to which are fastened two small bits of parchment shaped like the tip of the finger of a glove and sewed together in such a manner as that the food poured into the horn can be sucked through between the stitches. This appears to be a very simple and ingenious contrivance and is admired by some who look upon it as a kind of artificial nipple, and it might very well be considered as such if we had but the breast milk to convey through it. Or if we could discover any food of the same thinness with the milk, and as nourishing as it is, the horn might still answer.

But as a discovery of this kind is not to be expected, and the food which the child sucks through this artificial nipple must be thin in order to pass between the stitches, there requires a larger quantity to nourish the child, and hence its stomach and bowels are too much relaxed whereby it is in danger of falling into the watery gripes as was the case with two of mine which were fed for some time in this way ... The horn having succeeded so ill, I made no further trial of it, and the last child I had was fed with the boat ...

In 1777 Hugh Smith, author of *Letters to Married Women on Nursing and the Management of Children*, described a small pewter feeding vessel that was used 'by the Hollanders when they travel'. It was, he said, 'somewhat in the form of a cone which is filled with milk and a sponge covered with a linen cloth is tied over the smaller end. This serves the child very well as an artificial nipple.' In spite of the fact that the cloth-covered sponge must have been a constant source of gastro-intestinal troubles—one could hardly devise a more favourable breeding place for the bacteria contained in the milk—Hugh Smith contrived a milk-pot for his own nursery on more or less similar lines and obligingly allowed it to be used as a pattern for others:

... The model of this milk-pot is left with Mr Morrison at the Three Kings in Cheapside for the benefit of the pupils. The milk-pots are now also made in the Queens-ware [a type of stoneware manufactured by Messrs Wedgwood] in order that the public may be accommodated ...

As late as 1799, 'bubby-pots' of this kind were still being used by those who could afford them. In the following year, a book by C August Struve, originally published in 1798 in Hanover, appeared in an English translation. Called *A Compendium Addressed to all Mothers who are Seriously Concerned for the Welfare of their Offspring*, it contained one paragraph which suggests that an infant alive at that time might consider itself lucky if the unhygienic bubby-pot were all it had to contend with:

> ... One of the most disgusting customs is the sucking bag which is given to the child for the double purpose of nourishing and composing it. Many a poor mother will tear a rag from an old shirt or a clout which she has found perhaps in the street, and which may contain the remains of a venereal contagion: of this she makes a small bag, which is filled with bread, milk and sugar and then given to the child to suck. If the infant happens to drop this rag on the ground it is presented again though covered with dirt: a number of flies settle upon it when the child is alone which but the moment before may have quitted a saucer of poison ...

Not all mothers, during the eighteenth century, were seriously concerned for the welfare of their offspring. Far from it. Before even the seventeenth century was out, the well-to-do had found it convenient to farm out their babies, with poor women, for pay. Walter Harris, in his *De Morbis acutis infantum*, published in London in 1689, reported:

> ... The Rector of a Parish twelve miles from London with great grief of mind told me that his Parish which was not small either in its Bounds or Number of Inhabitants and was situated in a very Wholesome Air was, when he first came to it, filled with sucking Infants, and yet in the space of one Year that he had buried them all, except two and one of his own whom being weak he had happily committed to my Care from his very Birth, and that the same Number of Infants being soon twice supplied, according to the usual Custom of hireling Nurses, from the very great and almost inexhaustible City, he had

committed them all to their parent Earth in the very same Year . . .

By 1768 the appalling death rate among infants was causing (at last) some public concern. So, in that year, the members of the Committee of the Foundling Hospital in London decided to publish a treatise that had been sent anonymously to one of the Governors some years before. Entitled *An Essay upon Nursing and the Management of Children from their Birth to Three Years of Age. By a Physician*, the work went through a number of editions and had a profound influence on infant hygiene. The author—shown, eventually, to be a Doctor William Cadogan, of Bristol—was scathing about those ignorant enough to want to manage children according to the precepts of their great-grandmothers. If anyone wanted proof of the faulty character of the current mode of rearing children, Cadogan invited him to 'look over the Bills of Mortality, there he may observe that almost half the Number of those that fill up that Black List are under five Years of Age.' The author disapproved thoroughly of the prevalent habit of wet-nursing:

> . . . I am quite at a loss to account for the general Practice of sending Infants out of Doors to be suckled or dry-nursed by another Woman, who has not so much Understanding, nor can have so much Affection for it as the Parents: and how it comes to pass that People of good Sense and easy Circumstances will not give themselves the Pains to watch over the Health and Welfare of their Children: but are so careless as to give them up to the Common Methods, without considering how near it is to an equal Chance that they are destroyed by them. The ancient Custom of exposing them to wild Beasts or drowning them would certainly be a much quicker and more humane way of despatching them . . .

Doctor Cadogan was equally scathing about the prevalent practice of 'swaddling' very young children. From the remotest antiquity, midwives and children's nurses had believed that an infant would grow up distorted unless its body were moulded by the tightest bandaging directly it was born. François Mauriceau, whose book on obstetrics, published in France, was translated into English by Hugh Chamberlen the Elder, had repeated the fallacy:

> . . . Let his [the infant's] Arms and Legs be wrapped in his bed
> and stretched strait and swathed to keep them so, viz his Arms
> along his sides and his Legs equally both together with a little
> of the bed between them so that they may not be galled by
> rubbing one another: after all this the Head must be kept steady
> and strait with a stay fastned on each side the Blancket, and
> then wrap the Child up in Mantles or Blanckets to keep it warm.
> He must be thus swaddled to give his little body a strait Figure,
> which is most decent and convenient for a Man and to accustom
> him to keep upon the Feet, for else he would go upon all four
> as most other Animals do . . .

For several decades, Mauriceau's statement was accepted without
question by the midwives of Europe and America who used his
book as an instruction manual. Obediently, they and the mothers
they served swaddled their helpless little charges and they went
on doing so until William Cadogan poured scorn, publicly, on 'the
diabolical method of the nurses binding [the infants'] tender
bodies, as soon as born, with bandages so tight that the bowels nor
the limbs have any liberty to act and exert themselves in that free
easy way nature designed they should':

> . . . The first great Mistake is that they think a new-born
> Infant cannot be kept too warm: From this Prejudice they load
> it and bind it with Flannels, Wrappers, Swathes, Stays etc.
> commonly called Cloaths, which all together are almost equal to
> its own Weight . . .

Light, loose garments, said Cadogan:

> . . . Would be abundantly sufficient for the Day, laying aside
> all those swathes, bandages, stays and contrivances, that are
> most ridiculously used to close and keep the Head in its Place
> and support the Body, as if Nature, exact Nature, had produced
> her chief Work, a human Creature, so carelessly unfinished as
> to want those idle Aids to make it perfect. Shoes and Stockings
> are very needles Incumbrances, besides that they keep the Legs
> wet and nasty if they are not chang'd every Hour . . .

Until Cadogan made this revolutionary proposal, eighteenth-century infants—having their limbs tightly bound, and having an extraordinary mixture of unsuitable substances put into their stomachs—were very apt to suffer, as we have seen, from fits. Thomas Willis, leading physician in the city of London in the reign of King Charles II, graphically described these infantile paroxysms, and his account of them was still being reprinted in 1742 and studied on both sides of the Atlantic:

> ... Those convulsive Symptoms which frequently attack Infants soon after they are born, are Distortions of the Eyes, Distortions or Tremblings of the Cheeks and Lips, Contractions of the Tendons, Startings and sudden shakings of the Limbs, and often enough of the whole Body. Even the Viscera [bowels] seem not to be exempted from the Disease ...

The fits were caused by 'inordinate motion of the spirits in the brain', said Willis, and they could be cured by the use of a medicine:

> ... Take prepared Human Skull, Mistletoe of the Oak, Factitious Cinnabar, Elk's Hoof, of each Half an Ounce. Dose from ten Grains to a Scruple ...

Or by the use of a charm:

> ... An amulet made of the Roots and Seeds of Male Peony with a little Elk's Hoof should be hung about their [the little patients'] necks ...

Children were liable to suffer from the fits again about the time of teething, said Willis. Teething-time can bring its little worries for a child's parents even today. During the early part of the eighteenth century it was a critical period in a young person's development. Parents, then, who wanted to do something to relieve the agonies from which their offspring were apparently suffering were severely handicapped, since there had been no really new thinking on the subject for nearly two thousand years, and the old thinking was entirely misleading.

For Soranus of Ephesus, who lived in the first century AD, had declared positively that a hare's brain should be applied to the gums of a teething infant, if it were in pain, and would bring almost instant relief. Claudius Galen, who died in AD 200, had repeated this nonsense, and Oribasius, court physician and friend of the Emperor Julian, had repeated it yet again nearly two hundred years later. (Oribasius, though, suggested the use of dog's milk as a possible alternative.) There was scarcely a writer on the discomforts and diseases of children during the next fourteen hundred years who did not favour Soranus' original recommendation. (Some of these writers suggested that the hare's brains should be taken internally; a few thought that the brains would be equally effective used in either way.) François Mauriceau was one of the first medical men in any country to declare publicly that hares' brains were useless as a remedy in dentition, but his lack of enthusiasm for the ancient palliative was largely ignored.

In 1742 a small book appeared that dealt in simple and straightforward language with the problems of teething. (It was the first publication to be devoted exclusively to the subject since Hippocrates had produced a paper on it some four hundred years before the birth of Christ.) The modern work had an elegant if somewhat extended title. It was called:

A Practical Treatise upon Dentition or The Breeding of Teeth in Children, Wherein The Causes of the acute Symptoms arising in that dangerous Period are enquired into; The Remedies both of the Ancients and Moderns for the Cure of those Evils and the Prevention of their fatal Effects, are examined impartially; Some errors of Consequence corrected, Objections Answered; and A Right Practice recommended upon Observation and Experience. The whole illustrated with proper Cases and Remarks. By Joseph Hurlock, Surgeon

Joseph Hurlock, Surgeon, began his book with an attempt to show that teething was, at that time, one of the most fatal affections of infancy. In 1740, for instance, he said, the total deaths of those up to five years of age were 13,627, out of which 11,549 were attributed to 'convulsions, Smallpox and Teething' and he suggested that many of the convulsions that had unfortunately proved fatal were, themselves, due to troubles at teething. The figures he quoted cannot be regarded as conclusive, since, as he himself admitted, the causes of death were not certified at that time by properly qualified doctors. Instead, they were certified by uneducated women of the poorest class who were given the high-sounding title of 'Searchers'. A Searcher would report her views after a quick and superficial inspection of the corpse. More often than not, she would be wrong.

Although Joseph Hurlock had promised to examine the remedies both of the Ancients and Moderns impartially, it is clear from his book that he was a great believer in the efficacy of gum-lancing and had, in fact, embarked on his literary exercise largely in order to convert others to his views. The technique he wished to recommend had been described by the great French physician Ambroise Paré as long ago as 1597. Paré, said Hurlock, had seen gum-lancing, performed with a proper instrument, as a safer alternative to homelier but rougher methods:

> . . . Which kind of remedy is much better and more safe than to do as some Nurses do, who taught only by the instinct of Nature, with their nails and scratching, break and tear or rent the Childrens gums . . .

But gum-lancing must still have been regarded as a dangerous innovation in 1742 and Hurlock, plainly, had encountered a certain amount of opposition from his clients:

> . . . It is objected by some Parents that cutting the Gums of Infants is a novel Practice and a reason is demanded, Why they should not do as well now as heretofore without it? . . .

As Hurlock, in his book, describes cases in homes as far south of the centre of London as Southwark and as far north of it as Islington, as well as 'between Tottenham Road and Muswell Hill', he seems to have had a fairly extensive practice, in spite of these parental reservations. And he was not afraid to put his beliefs to the test in his own home. When his first-born daughter, in her infancy, had a convulsion:

... I quickly catch'd her up, took an instrument from my Pocket and immediately opened her Gums, apprehending this evil from Back-teeth. *In the very instant of cutting* the Gum she opened her eyes wide ... And all the convulsive Symptoms of this first fit disappeared ...

One small child Hurlock had been called to see was ' ... under great Trouble from his Teeth crying in a violent manner and not able to sleep ... ' True to his usual form, Hurlock lanced the small sufferer's gums. Then, as the little patient was 'loose in its bowels', it occurred to him to enquire 'into the Order of Diet', whereupon he was told by the child's mother that 'she gave him anything he liked, such as Meat, Cheese, Strong Liquors, and Cucumbers in a large quantity, and that he would eat Pepper with these to a degree hardly to be credited!'

Where general hygiene is poor, intestinal parasites usually abound, especially in the young. Worms are a major problem in the developing countries today. They were an unrelenting scourge in the eighteenth century. Nils Rosen von Rosenstein, brilliant Swedish pædiatrician and author of the classic *Diseases of Children and their Remedies*, which was published in Stockholm in 1765 and in London eleven years later, described five different types of worm that plagued the human young in that uncomfortable period of history. He added:

... All these five sorts of worms, I fancy, will seldom be found in one person. But I know a poor man's child of four years old, who was very lean and weak: on receiving a little dram of barleybrandy from the mother as a cordial, it immediately after voided an innumerable quantity of ascarides [thread worms], eight feet of a slender tape worm, and ten worms of the second and fourth sort. These guests being expelled, the child recovered strength and a jolly appearance ...

Here is part of von Rosenstein's charming pen-picture of the tape worm:

... When a tape worm first comes out, it is always something longer and broader than a little afterwards; one can also observe a reptile motion in it when it is expelled alive, how it alternately grows broader and more narrow, and that the edges of it are tumbled as it were like waves; and that is the tumbling or undulating motion patients complain of who are infected by this worm. One would sometimes think it quite dead after being expelled, though it is still alive. I have frequently tried this even after its having laid on a plate in the window for twenty-four hours; for when I put it into a bowl, and poured on it some warm water, its creepings and motions were immediately to be observed, but on pouring a little cold water on it again, the motions ceased, and the worm appeared to be dead; and in this manner I repeatedly could make it torpid and revivified again . . .

No one who had worms could be secure for a single moment from being attacked by them, said von Rosenstein. Anything that could possibly cause the worms to move, creep, suck, or try to bore their way through the intestines (as, for example, if the host ate something sweet, or some unaccustomed kind of food) would immediately bring on sickness or discomfort. Worms were especially active at the time of the waning of the moon, he went on, and at the very beginning of its increase. The ascarides worm was—according to this expert—really troublesome only in the evenings.

The easiest way to 'worm' a child was, obviously, to give it a strong laxative. Von Rosenstein recommended that the little sufferer should be persuaded to eat raw carrots. Alternatively, he said, it should be made to drink birch juice, or it should suck the juice from the bark of a young fir tree until 'a looseness' was produced. Less humane eighteenth-century authorities than von Rosenstein prescribed much more violent purgatives.

A little more difficult to administer than a worming laxative was a 'clyster' or enema, since this had to be inserted into the small patient by means of a hollow pipe or tube at the other end of the alimentary canal. Among the clysters recommended by von Rosenstein for the eradication of worms was a solution of salt in tepid milk. Another of his favourite clysters was one made by adding to tepid milk equal quantities of fine sugar and rats' dung, the two solids having previously been well rubbed together.

Tobacco smoke, said von Rosenstein, made the best worming clyster of all.

A sporting element was introduced into child-worming by yet another technique recommended by the great Swedish pioneer. In this, a string was tied to a piece of fresh pork, and the bait was then introduced into the *intestinum rectum* of the small sufferer. After a short time, the meat would be pulled out again and (hopefully) a number of the ever-hungry worms would follow. The process should be repeated with fresh pieces of pork, von Rosenstein recommended, until all the worms had been evacuated.

'The Rickets' affected almost as many children in some parts of Europe during the eighteenth century as worms. The 'Famous Emporium of England, London' was specially apt to produce and foster the disease, said Friedrich Hofmann, of Halle (1660–1742) in one of the earliest books ever to be devoted entirely to the diseases of the young. The proneness of Londoners to become rickety was not only on account of the moisture given off by the surrounding sea, he said, but it was due, too, to the particles given off by the enormous quantities of coal burned in the Thames-side city. Like so many other eighteenth-century medical theoreticians who were sure they were right, Hofmann was just about as wrong as he could have been.

Called, sometimes, 'Doubling of the Joints', and, at other times, 'Tent', this distressing condition had probably been recognized for centuries by members of the lay public and may even have been discussed in medical circles, but it was not specifically mentioned in medical literature until 1645, when it was described for the first time by one of the students at Leyden University who was writing a thesis for his Doctor of Medicine degree. (This student, named Daniel Whistler, later became President of the College of Physicians in London, and a close friend of Samuel Pepys. He was mentioned, typically, in the latter's diary: 'Two daughters of Dr Whistler's with whom I and Creed had mighty sport at supper, the ladies very pretty and mirthfull . . . ') Whistler advanced the theory that the name most often given to the disease by the English—'The Rickets'—was derived from the surname of some quack called Ricket or Rickett who had been the first to treat it.

'Who had been the first to *try* to treat it,' it would be more accurate to say, for the disease baffled everyone. Enlargement of the liver was one of its preliminary symptoms—that was generally agreed in medical circles—and this was followed by enlargement of the head, by weakness and wasting of the limbs, by curvature of the spine, and, eventually, by a complete inability of the sufferer to stand up at all. How, though, was such a progressive and incapacitating decline to be halted? No two 'experts' could agree about that.

Francis Glisson, who published a treatise on the disease in London just six years after Daniel Whistler gave his important thesis to the professors at Leyden, recommended for sufferers from 'The Rickets' various simples, which included 'Earthworms, the Livers of Frogs and young Ravens, Woodlice washt in white wine, bak'd in an Oven and beaten to powder and such like things', but these would obviously be ineffective. They went on being prescribed, though, well into the eighteenth century.

By 1746 the fact that there might be some connection between dietary deficiencies and 'The Rickets' had at last been noticed. It was 'a Distemper extremely common in London', repeated Jean Astruc, Professor of Medicine at Paris, in a treatise translated into English in that year. As there were many people in that city who fed their infants on water-pap only, he added, and gave them no milk of any kind, this was scarcely to be wondered at. This important clue to the possible causes of the disease was for many years almost entirely ignored by the members of the medical profession. So, it was not until long after the end of the eighteenth century that the problems of 'The Rickets' were satisfactorily solved. The caricatures of Thomas Rowlandson (1756–1827) are plentifully furnished with the disease's distorted victims. (In some of his pictures, the twisted and crippled seem to outnumber those more normally developed.)

'Thrush', like 'The Rickets', has practically disappeared from our contemporary scene. Very prevalent in the eighteenth century, it was a revolting disease which would bring up parasitic fungoid growths in a child's mouth and throat. Caused, generally, by a combination of malnutrition and dirtiness, the thrush growths, when they appeared, were often treated lightly by the negligent mothers and nurses who were largely responsible. 'Everyone has to have Thrush once in their life,' these ignorant females would excuse themselves readily, 'either at birth or at death. Better to get it over and done with now.'

There were several infectious diseases—smallpox, the typhus and typhoid fevers, the measles and diphtheria among them—that destroyed infants and children in eighteenth-century epidemics almost as rapidly as wildfire can eradicate dry stubble. (Out of 300 children affected by an outbreak of smallpox in Sweden, 270 died, according to von Rosenstein.) As these diseases were liable to attack adults, too, they will be dealt with in Chapter 4. Whooping cough, though not so generally fatal, was —and is—primarily a disease of the young. So this distressing infantile complaint must find its place with the nursery disorders.

'The fevers attacked children of four months, ten months, and a little older, and carried off an enormous number,' wrote Guillaume de Baillou, Dean of the Faculty of Medicine in the University of Paris, describing an epidemic that had occurred in that city in 1578. 'Especially that common cough which is popularly called Quinta or Quintana ... The symptoms of this are severe. The lung is so irritated that in its struggle to drive out by utmost effort the cause of irritation, it can neither inspire, nor with any ease expire. The patient seems to swell up, and as if on the verge of suffocation with his breathing obstructed in mid throat ... '

De Baillou was unable to explain why whooping cough had been dubbed 'Quinta' and 'Quintana'. The words might have been derived from the choking noise young people make when they suffer from the cough, he suggested. Alternatively, they might have come from some Latin name given to the cough because it tended to recur at intervals of (approximately) five hours. Between the crises, he said, a sufferer was frequently quite free from distress. When the paroxysms returned, they would sometimes be so violent that blood would be driven out from the patient's mouth and nose.

Treating the whooping cough, in the seventeenth and eighteenth centuries, was, like so much other therapeutic work carried out at the time, a matter of making shots in the dark. Some physicians, believing that the cough was caused by a disordered flux of the humours from the brain to the lungs, covered their little patients' heads with flannel cowls. (The heat engendered, they thought, would draw the errant humours back to their normal and proper seat.) Other physicians prescribed belladonna, syrup of poppies with oxymel of squills, or 'Jesuit's Bark'. (The medicinal value of Cinchona, from which quinine is produced, was known to the Jesuits at Lima by about 1630, hence its popular name, and the alternative name 'Peruvian Bark'. After the evil-tasting substance was introduced into Europe its effectiveness was quickly recognized and it was soon used to treat all kinds of illness. Lady Cave, writing to Lord Fermanagh about her nephew Tommy, said 'He has taken three quarts of Bark and is to go on with it longer, so I hope he'll pick up again'.)

Few of the medicines prescribed for whooping cough prior to the nineteenth century seem to have been worth taking. Even the grand and enormously prosperous Thomas Willis, Doctor of Medicine, whose monument in London's Westminster Abbey records that 'the world itself would scarce suffice to hold his praise', admitted publicly that he found the Quinta very difficult to cure. 'The plan of treatment which is usual in other varieties of cough is seldom of any use in this,' he wrote in 1675. 'Which is the reason why old women and gypsies are consulted more often than doctors.' If all orthodox preparations fail, he said, the shock of a sudden fright might stop the whooping. He could do no better than that.

More than a hundred years later, 'the shock of a sudden fright' was still being publicly extolled. In 1781 Doctor William Moss of Liverpool, who was very conscious of the absurdity of many of the remedies being prescribed by his more fashionable rivals, said of the whooping cough:

> . . . When the complaint takes a favourable turn it is frequently attributed to the means that were last used: hence that means is ever after recorded as infallible. As it is a disease of the spasmodic or convulsive kind it has been sometimes relieved, or even removed, by a shock or sudden fright: thus riding upon a bear (a frightful mode of travelling no doubt) from the fright it occasions has been said to be serviceable. Giving the patient a part of some disgraceful animal, as a mouse, &c, to eat, and afterwards informing him of it; and so forth . . .

Not all the sick children treated gratuitously to a shock or sudden fright came out unscathed from the experience. In the *Gentleman's Magazine* of Wednesday, 25 August 1736, it was reported that two remarkable trials had 'come on' at Rochester, in the County of Kent:

> ... One ... of a Soldier who pretended to cure a Boy of an Ague, and thinking to frighten it away, by firing his Piece over the Boy's Head, levell'd it too low, and shot his Brains out ...

The soldier, modern liberals may be glad to hear, was found Not Guilty, and was acquitted.

It is always darkest—the proverb *must* be repeated—just before the dawn. The horrors that infants and children went through (or failed to survive) during the eighteenth century scarcely bear repeating. But just before the century ended, the faintest glimmer of light appeared above the horizon. William Buchan, in a book called *Domestic Medicine* published in 1769, had recommended that girls should be specially trained in the care of children so that they should not be totally incapable when they, in their turn, had infants to cherish and protect:

> ... It is indeed to be regretted that more care is not bestowed in teaching the proper management of children to those whom Nature has designed for mothers. This instead of being made the principle is seldom considered as any part of female education. Is it any wonder when females so educated come to be mothers, that they should be quite ignorant of the duties belonging to that character? However strange it may appear it is certainly true that many mothers, and those of fashion too, are as ignorant, when they have a child into the world, what to do for it as the infant itself ...

Doctor Tytler who, in 1798, published a translation of a very learned work about children's diseases, took William Buchan's idea and carried it a stage or two further. Girls, he said, 'might be trained to the proper management of children if a premium were given in free schools, workhouses, etc, to those that brought up the finest child to one year old.' Social conditions were slowly starting to alter, then. The eighteenth century, which saw at its start the most callous indifference to the sufferings of infants, ended with the first public admissions that the hand that rocked the cradle (and, therefore, ruled the world) was not doing its job very well.

5

Some Fevers
and Infectious Diseases

... Here, where men sit and hear each other groan,
Where youth grows pale, and spectre-thin, and dies ...

JOHN KEATS, 1795–1821

In the seventeenth and eighteenth centuries, the word 'plague' was applied loosely to any epidemic fever that caused large numbers of those affected to die. Today, we use the name a little more precisely, to describe, specifically, the fevers caused by the *bacillus pestis*. Of these, the bubonic plague is one of the most deadly.

The great cycle of epidemics which, in the fourteenth century, carried away approximately half the adult population of Britain is referred to, now, as the 'Black Death'. Some, if not all, of those fatal epidemics were undoubtedly visitations of the bubonic plague. When the members of any impoverished community are forced to share their dwellings with rats and with the fleas with which those rats will inevitably be infested, those poor people will be liable to suffer from that appalling disease, which causes the glands to swell agonizingly, until the pain becomes a torture that can no longer be borne. Death from the bubonic plague is rated, with crucifixion, among the nastiest human experiences of all.

In the years 1664 and 1665, rat-infested London suffered a visitation from the Great Plague. Rich citizens and poor citizens alike were defenceless against the scourge. Pits were dug and filled quickly with the heaped bodies of those who had been infected by the evil and had succumbed. After that, there were no really serious epidemics of bubonic plague in Britain, though single cases occurred sporadically until 1679, when the disease appeared to die out altogether. (In 1703, it was reckoned that the word 'plague' could be safely omitted from the mortality returns.) There were isolated epidemics after that in Germany in 1707 and in France in 1720, but these seemed, as far as Western Europe was concerned, like the last flickerings of a fire that had blazed too fiercely and had burned itself out.

Disappearance of the plague from London was generally attributed to the Great Fire of 1666, but no such cause could be produced for the disappearance of the disease from other cities. Quarantine has also been suggested, but no effective quarantine was established in England until 1720, so the dying-out of the plague in Britain must be considered as having been spontaneous. The similar disappearance of the plague noted shortly afterwards in the greater part of Western Europe appears also to have been spontaneous.

Though they appeared to have been freed from the ravages of the plague, the people of Britain and all neighbouring countries were still liable to fall victim to other deadly infectious diseases. Among these, one of the most dreaded during the late seventeenth and eighteenth centuries was smallpox—'the most terrible of all the ministers of death', in Lord Macaulay's words. The smallpox, he said, was always present:

> ... Filling the churchyards with corpses, tormenting with constant fears all whom it had not yet stricken, leaving on those whose lives it spared the hideous traces of its power, turning the babe into a changeling at which the mother shuddered, and making the eyes and cheeks of the betrothed maiden objects of horror to the lover ...

Smallpox was a nauseating disease. Fortunately, it has so nearly disappeared from the face of the earth that the use of the present tense, in describing it, would hardly seem appropriate. Those unlucky enough to suffer from it would, almost inevitably, be covered with nasty eruptions. These eruptions would usually appear first on the face, particularly about the forehead and the roots of the hair, and they would take the form of dusky red spots which would develop, in the course of a few hours, into true 'papules', or clusters of pimples more or less thickly grouped together.

Then, these disfigurements would spread, during the next few hours, over the whole of the patient's face, trunk and extremities. The painful swellings they produced in the mucous membranes of the mouth could be an acute source of danger, since they tended to cause serious obstructions in the upper air passages. If they occurred on or near the eyes, they were liable to cause permanent blindness.

On the second or third day after the papules appeared, they would change into bladder-like 'vesicles', which would be filled with a clear liquid. Then, gradually, this liquid would cloud, and pustules would form. As this happened, the skin would swell so much, and would become so inflamed, that the patient's features would often be almost unrecognizable. Frequently, the sufferer, at this stage of the disease, would be delirious.

On the eleventh or twelfth day—if the patient had survived that long—the pustules would begin to dry up and a great itching of the skin would provide additional torment. Gradually, then, the scabs produced by the dried pustules would drop off, leaving behind them, as permanent disfigurements, the ugly white depressed scars or craters referred to by Lord Macaulay.

Towards the end of the year 1694, there were even more cases of smallpox than usual in London. The infection spread at length to the royal out-of-town residence at Kensington, and it reached, eventually, Mary, the pious and devoted wife of King William III. For two or three days the queen felt poorly, as most people do from time to time. Her pulse raced. She had a splitting headache. She vomited, more than once. She had pains in her loins and back. Would she have been better off, her ladies-in-waiting wondered, in the damper but less remote royal apartments in riverside Westminster?

Then, more serious symptoms appeared. Sir Thomas Millington, who was physician in ordinary to the king, thought that the queen had caught the measles. John Radcliffe, a man of humble origin who, in spite of his coarse and overbearing manners and ignorance of book learning had built up the largest and most profitable practice in London, chiefly by his rare skill in diagnosing, thought otherwise. Radcliffe, observing that the dusky red spots on poor Mary's royal brow were turning into the universally dreaded pustules, uttered the terrifying words 'It could be smallpox . . . '

The queen received the news that she was in the gravest danger with true greatness of soul, according to Lord Macaulay. She gave orders that every lady of her bedchamber, every maid of honour—even, every menial servant—who had not had the smallpox should instantly leave Kensington House. She locked herself up for a short while in her own room, destroyed some papers, arranged others, and then calmly awaited her fate. Within a few days, William was ruling alone.

Queen Mary had been dead for more than twenty years before anyone in Western Europe had even the slightest hint that the dreadful and ever-present scourge of smallpox might be eliminated. The hint came from the remarkable Lady Mary Wortley Montagu.

Lady Mary was born in 1689. She was the eldest daughter of Evelyn Pierrepont, an autocratic landowner who became in 1690 the fifth Earl of Kingston and in 1706 was created the first Marquis of Dorchester. When she was barely out of the schoolroom, Lady Mary met, and was immediately attracted to, Edward Wortley Montagu, a man of ability and some scholarship who had represented Huntingdon in the House of Commons since 1705. Montagu, on his part, was equally impressed by the girl's wit and beauty as well as by her knowledge of Latin.

Soon, Montagu told Lord Dorchester that he wished to marry his daughter. It seemed at first sight an excellent match, but when Montagu, who disapproved on principle of marriage settlements, refused to entail his estates on the first son of the alliance, Lord Dorchester showed him the door and ordered his daughter to marry someone else who would be a little more tractable.

So, settlements were duly drawn up for the girl's marriage to the more amenable 'other man', and the wedding date was fixed. Before the day arrived, however, Lady Mary stole quietly out of the house and married Montagu privately, by special licence.

That elopement was to play an important part in the history of preventive medicine, for, in June 1716, Montagu was appointed ambassador to the Porte, then at war with Austria. The embassy was intended to reconcile the Turks and the Emperor. Montagu left London with his wife at the end of July and, after a slow journey across Europe and into the Near East, reached Adrianople early in the following year. Lady Mary's interest in the manners of the countries through which she passed is shown by the many and brilliant letters in which she recorded her impressions. In a letter written at Adrianople on 1 April 1717, she reported the practice of inoculation for the prevention of smallpox:

... I am going to tell you a thing that I am sure will make you wish yourself here.

The smallpox, so fatal and so general among us, is here rendered entirely harmless by the invention of ingrafting, which is the term they give it. There is a set of old women who make it their business to perform the operation every autumn, in the month of September, when the great heat is abated. People send to one another to know if any of their family has a mind to have the smallpox; they make parties for this purpose, and when they are met (commonly fifteen or sixteen together), the old woman comes with a nutshell full of the matter of the best sort of smallpox, and asks what veins you please to have opened. She immediately rips open that you offer to her with a large needle (which gives you no more pain than a common scratch), and puts into the vein as much venom as can lie upon the head of her needle, and after binds up the little wound with a hollow bit of shell; and in this manner opens four or five veins. The Grecians have commonly the superstition of opening one in the middle of the forehead, in each arm, and on the breast to mark the sign of the cross; but this has a very ill effect, all these wounds leaving little scars, and it is not done by those that are not superstitious, who choose to have them in the legs, or that part of the arm that is concealed. The children or young patients play together all the rest of the day, and are in perfect health to the eighth. Then the fever begins to seize them, and they keep their beds two days, very seldom three. Every year thousands undergo this operation; and the French ambassador says pleasantly, that they take the smallpox here by way of diversion, as they take the waters in other countries.

There is no example of anyone that has died in it; and you may well believe I am very well satisfied of the safety of this experiment, since I intend to try it on my dear little son ...

Lady Mary did have inoculation tried on her dear little son, and after the family returned to England at the end of October 1718 she went to a lot of trouble to make other people aware of the advantages of the operation. Under her distinguished and energetic patronage, a Mr Maitland, who had been the physician of her husband's embassy, started to carry out the first British inoculations. By 1721 the possibilities of protection offered by the newly imported practice had been successfully demonstrated, and the services of Mr Maitland were in ever-increasing demand.

Other physicians, inevitably, followed Mr Maitland's lead. Prominent among them was Claudius Amyand, who was the second son of another Huguenot refugee. Having been appointed Serjeant-Surgeon to King George I, Amyand was in an especially favourable position to act as an advocate for the new technique.

Hearing inoculation recommended warmly and volubly by her friend Lady Mary Wortley Montagu and by her royal father-in-law's Serjeant-Surgeon Mr Amyand, Princess Caroline, wife of the future King George II, decided that her own children ought, properly, to be protected against smallpox by the recently-introduced method. Before she took the great step, however, she persuaded the king to allow experimental inoculations to be carried out on six prisoners in Newgate Gaol who had been condemned to death. The men agreed to undergo the operation on being told that if they survived it, they would be pardoned. Five of the criminals recovered. The sixth kept very quiet about the fact that he had previously suffered from smallpox and, therefore, would not be affected anyway. So, all six men avoided the gallows. In the following spring, the Princess of Wales directed that a number of poor pupils at a charity school should also be inoculated by Claudius Amyand. None of the children died, so the Serjeant-Surgeon was ordered to 'engraft the smallpox' on the Princess Amelia, aged eleven, and the Princess Caroline, aged nine.

When the little princesses, in their turn, came through their ordeal successfully, inoculation became all the rage. Steele praised Lady Mary highly in a paper in the *Plain Dealer*, congratulating her on her 'godlike delight' of saving many thousands of British lives every year. One of the busiest 'engrafters'—Thomas Dimsdale, of Hertford, to the north of London—was summoned to Russia in 1768 to inoculate the Empress Catherine the Great and her son. He received, for his trouble, a fee of £10,000, a yearly pension of £500, and a barony.

In spite of all this international acclaim, smallpox inoculation had certain pronounced drawbacks. In some instances—regardless of all Lady Mary's protestations about its safety—it brought on the disease in an unalleviated form. In other instances, it caused the person inoculated to pass on the disease to other people. Quite frequently these unpremeditated consequences proved fatal. It was Edward Jenner—as every schoolchild used to know—who found, at last, a way of preventing smallpox that was just as simple as the Turkish method, but which was very much safer.

Jenner was born in 1749 in the village of Berkeley, in the West of England, and was brought up there. The village, built almost in the shadow of historic Berkeley Castle, stands in rich farmland, where great numbers of cows and horses were, and are, kept. While he was a boy there, Jenner became aware of the disease known to the local farmers and farriers as 'cowpox' and 'the grease'.

A cow suffering from cowpox, Jenner saw, would develop irregularly shaped pustules or ulcers on its teats. Then it would lose condition rapidly and its milk yield would drop. Before it had ceased to need milking altogether, it would probably have passed on the disease to the milkmaid whose hands had been squeezing its swollen and discoloured nipples.

Poor milkmaid! Inflamed spots would soon start to appear on various parts of her hands, and on her wrists, and before long these spots—roughly circular, and of a colour distantly approaching blue—would probably be exuding pus in an uncomfortable and unsightly fashion. From her, the infection would spread to the other domestics on the farm and, possibly, to the master and mistress. Before the trouble moved away, every human on the holding might well have suffered the unpleasant consequences of the cowpox.

Unpleasant consequences, yes . . . But not (in eighteenth-century terms) disastrous consequences. The humans affected would have a few aches and pains, and their pulses might race. They would shiver occasionally, or feel extra-hot, and they might be sick two or three times . . . But, they would not *die* . . . And, three or four days later, they would be as well as they had ever been. Moreover, it was said locally that dairymaids who had suffered the minor discomforts of the cowpox had never been known to suffer, later, from the much more dreaded smallpox.

When he was old enough to do so, Jenner went to be apprenticed to a surgeon named Daniel Ludlow, at Sodbury, near Bristol. Then, in 1770, he moved to London to be a pupil of the celebrated John Hunter. During his time in the capital, he was invited by Sir Joseph Banks to prepare and arrange the zoological specimens that Banks had collected on Captain Cook's first voyage of discovery in 1771. He did this so efficiently that he was offered the post of naturalist in Cook's second expedition. Preferring to practise his profession in his native county, Jenner declined the offer and returned to Berkeley, little more than three years after he had left the place.

There followed, for Jenner, a period of restless mental activity. Besides studying the geology of the district in which he lived, and such extraordinary phenomena as the breeding habits of the cuckoo, he helped to construct, in his spare time, the first aerial balloon ever seen in that part of the world. Of more relevance to his profession, he helped to found a medical society which used to hold meetings at the Fleece Inn, Rodborough. At these meetings, the members would read papers on medical subjects and would dine afterwards. Jenner—it is known—read memoirs on angina pectoris, ophthalmia and valvular disease of the heart, and sometimes raised the question of inoculation for smallpox, making remarks about cowpox, which was already engaging his attention.

For some years, then, it would be safe to say, the idea of vaccination was germinating slowly in Jenner's mind. Then, in 1794, he had typhus fever severely, and after he recovered he began to research intensively into the cowpox-smallpox question.

At first, he worked up a blind alley, studying 'the grease'—a disease mentioned earlier, which affected horses, causing inflammation and swelling in the animals' hocks. Could cowpox be caused by male farm servants who, after dressing the hocks of diseased horses, were required to help with the milking, he wondered? He came to the conclusion that cowpox and 'the grease' were one and the same disease. He has since been shown, conclusively, to have been wrong.

He moved on to surer ground in May 1796. On the fourteenth day of that month, he took a specially selected healthy boy, about eight years old, named James Phipps. Then he took some lymph from a cowpox sore on the hand of a dairymaid called Sarah Nelmes, who had been infected by one of her master's cows, and he inserted this into the arm of the boy, making, for the purpose, two superficial cuts, each about an inch long, that barely penetrated the cuticle.

Seven days after this, the boy complained of some uneasiness in the armpit.

On the ninth day, young James became 'a little chilly'; he lost his appetite; he had a slight headache. During the whole of this day—observed Jenner—the boy was perceptibly indisposed. He spent the night 'with some degree of restlessness'. On the following day, Jenner was enormously relieved to find that the boy was feeling perfectly well. The scabs that had formed on the vaccinated parts came away, eventually, without giving Jenner or his young patient the slightest trouble.

Next, Jenner had to find out if the boy, after suffering so little from the introduction into his system of the cowpox virus, was secure from the contagion of the smallpox proper.

To do this, he inoculated young James, on the first day of the following July, with lymph taken directly from the pustules of someone suffering from smallpox. Jenner made several slight punctures and incisions on both the boy's arms and he inserted the possibly fatal matter with the utmost care.

No disease followed.

Several months afterwards, Jenner again inoculated the boy with 'live' smallpox lymph.

Again—to use Jenner's own words—'no sensible effect was produced on the constitution'. Jenner, then, was certain that his reasoning was correct.

Some of the notes Jenner made, in his own hand, about his momentous experiments are carefully preserved now at the Royal College of Surgeons in London, and are endorsed by the writer 'On the Cow-pox, the original paper'. The notes end with the words 'I shall endeavour still further to prosecute this inquiry, an inquiry I trust not merely speculative, but of sufficient moment to inspire the pleasing hope of its becoming essential to mankind'.

Those notes were never printed, but in June 1798 Jenner published, in London, a fuller account of his observations and conclusions. This short treatise, which will always be regarded as one of the classics of medical literature, was called *An Inquiry into the Cause and Effects of the Variolae Vaccinae, a Disease discovered in some of the Western Counties of England, particularly Gloucestershire, and known by the name of the Cow-pox.*

The booklet, seventy-five pages long, was dedicated to Doctor C H Parry, of Bath. It contained some coloured plates, one of which showed the hand of Sarah Nelmes, disfigured with vaccine pustules. Twenty-three separate cases were described, and Jenner announced, at the end, this important conclusion: 'The cow-pox protects the human constitution from the infection of small-pox.'

During all the early summer of 1798, Jenner stayed in London, attempting to bring his great discovery to the attention of the medical world. He suffered one real disappointment—in the capital, he could find no one who would allow himself, or herself, to be vaccinated.

About a month after he returned to the sweet green fields of Gloucestershire, a Mr Cline, who was a surgeon at St Thomas's Hospital, vaccinated some patients with lymph provided by Jenner. Having observed the results, Cline tried to persuade Jenner to settle permanently in London and assured his colleague from the west that he would earn a very large income in a metropolitan practice. Jenner wrote back from Berkeley to say that he had had quite enough of London. He preferred to live in the country.

During the next few years, then, Jenner continued his researches at Berkeley and at Cheltenham, replying patiently and at some length to those who had doubts about his innovations. Slowly, the practice of vaccination gained ground. In February 1800, Jenner was invited to stay at Petworth, Lord Egremont's great mansion in Sussex, and while he was there he vaccinated nearly two hundred of the local people with great success. In the following month, he was presented by Lord Berkeley to King George III and the king graciously accepted the dedication of the second edition of the *Inquiry*. All appeared to be going well, but there were occasional setbacks when vaccinations went wrong

through being carelessly carried out by inexperienced practitioners. More than once, the fluid from smallpox pustules was used,
in error, instead of the lymph from cowpox.

Quite soon after the publication of Jenner's *Inquiry*, news of his
great discovery started to travel abroad. Doctor Benjamin Waterhouse, Professor of Physic at Cambridge, Massachusetts, who
received from his friend Doctor Lettsom of London a copy of
Jenner's 'elegant publication', sent an account of the English
doctor's experiments with the cowpox to the *Columbian Sentinel*,
and it was printed in that paper on 12 March 1799 under the
eye-catching heading 'Something Curious in the Medical Line'.
Conceiving it his public duty to experiment further, Waterhouse
sent letters to England, asking for some of the cowpox matter, for
trial. After several fruitless attempts, he obtained some from
Jenner 'by a short passage from Bristol', and with it he inoculated
all the younger members of his family.

Waterhouse's experiments were, in the main, successful, but
(as had previously occurred in Britain), in a few subsequent
American cases lymph taken from smallpox pustules was used,
by mistake, instead of cowpox fluid, and the disease was thus
helped to spread, instead of being checked. Again, this was only a
temporary setback. By 1801 all the sailors of the British fleet were
being vaccinated. Soon, vaccination was known and was being
recommended by most doctors in all parts of the civilized world.

During the early part of the eighteenth century, Britain's
American colonists were seriously troubled by severe epidemics of
measles. The disease had been well described by Thomas Syden-
ham, as early as 1670:

> ... These Measles began very early, as they were wont to do,
> viz at the beginning of January ... and increasing daily, came
> to their height in March: afterwards they gradually decreased
> and were quite extinguish'd in the following July ...

The diary of Cotton Mather, of Massachusetts, provides a grim
picture of one of these epidemics. Mather, father of fifteen children, only two of whom survived him, lost three of his children
and his wife in the space of less than two weeks in the great
measles outbreak of 1713:

... For these many Months [he wrote] and ever since I heard of the venemous Measles invading the Countrey sixty Miles to the Southward of us, I have had a strong Distress on my Mind, that it will bring on my poor Family, a Calamity, which is now going to be inflicted. I have often, often express'd my Fear unto my Friends concerning it. And now, *the Thing that I greatly feared is coming upon me!*

When I saw my Consort safely delivered, and very easy, and the Measles appearing with favourable Symptomes upon her, and the Physician apprehending all to look very comfortably, I flattered myself, that my Fear was all over.

But this Day we are astonished, at the surprising Symptomes of Death upon her; after an extreme Want of Rest by Sleep, for diverse whole Dayes and Nights together.

To part with so desireable, so agreeable a Companion, a Dove from such a Nest of young ones too! Oh! the sad Cup, which my Father has appointed me! I now see the Meaning and the Reason of it, that I have never yett been able to make any Work of it, in Prayers and Cries to God, that such a Cup as this might pass from me. My Supplications have all along had, a most unaccountable Death and Damp upon them!

Tho' my dear Consort, had been so long without Sleep, yett she retained her Understanding.

I had and us'd my Opportunities as well as I could, continually to be assisting her, with Discourses that might support her in this Time, and prepare her for what was now before us ...

... Much weakness continues on some of my other Children. Especially the Eldest. And the poor Maid in the Family, is very like to dy ...

Diphtheria was not given its present name until 1826, but we can be reasonably sure that under some other descriptive title or titles this excruciating and dangerous disease was raging round Europe for at least three centuries before that date. (An epidemic of some choking throat disease that broke out in Nuremberg in 1492 was almost certainly diphtheria.) At the end of the sixteenth century, it was causing some exquisite suffering in Spain, where it was called 'garrotillo' after the nationally-favoured method of execution by strangling. In 1610, there were outbreaks of diphtheria in Italy. The disease appears to have crossed the Atlantic shortly after that, for cases were reported at Roxbury, Massachusetts, in 1659. Then it attacked the American Indians who, for some unknown reason, seem to have been particularly vulnerable. Samuel Bard, whose name will always be associated with the foundation in 1768 of King's College, New York, wrote, three years after the college opened, an *Essay on the Angina Suffocativa* which was hailed as a classic of medical literature. Regrettably, in spite of all Bard's cleverness, the victims of diphtheria continued to be strangled and to suffocate, and the disease still causes a certain amount of trouble today.

Almost as much dreaded as the epidemics of smallpox, measles and diphtheria, during the eighteenth century, were the recurrent visitations of the infectious diseases we know now as 'typhus' and 'typhoid fever'.

Two hundred and fifty years ago these diseases were still generally referred to as 'The Pests', as they had been for some centuries before.

No difference was seen between 'The Low Contagious Fevers'— another popular name for typhus and typhoid—until the eighteenth century was nearly half-way through. Then, one Doctor John Huxham of Totnes, in Devon, who had been a pupil of Hermann Boerhaave at Leyden, was able to study at first hand a particularly virulent outbreak of the fevers that laid low most of the seamen in the nearby dockyard at Plymouth. As a result of his observations, Huxham was able to publish, in 1755, an *Essay on Fevers*, in which he drew a particular distinction between the 'slow nervous fever' (*febris nervosa lente*) and the 'putrid malignant fever' (*febris putrida*).

We call the 'slow nervous fever', today, 'typhoid' or 'enteric' fever. The onset of this distressing disorder is, as the name Huxham gave it implies, less sudden than that of most other fevers, but its comparatively benign approach is deceptive, for typhoid fever can all too easily prove fatal—from internal bleeding, or from exhaustion. In the former case, an ulcer caused by the disease in the wall of the intestine will probably have perforated, resulting in sudden and intense abdominal pain, together with vomiting and signs of collapse. In the eighteenth century, a disaster of this kind would lead almost inevitably to peritonitis and, subsequently, to the death of the patient. As the disease is usually disseminated through the pollution of soil, food and drink—particularly milk and water—typhoid fever was, in that unhygienic century, one of the least easily avoidable hazards of human existence.

Typhus fever—called, by Huxham, the 'putrid malignant fever'—has been known in epidemic form in different parts of the world for tens of centuries. On the fourth or fifth day of the fever —occasionally, a little later—dark red spots or blotches appear on the sufferer's abdomen, back and sides and, in certain cases, on the patient's face. Delirium is normally present both by night and day. Usually, the feverish person mutters away quietly to himself or herself, but in severe cases the patient may behave wildly, or even like a maniac, in which case he or she will have to be subdued. In one peculiar condition associated with the typhus, the sufferer, though quite unconscious, lies with his or her eyes wide open, but unseeing. In the eighteenth century this state—known then as the 'coma vigil'—inevitably foretold the coming of death.

We know, now, that typhus fever is spread, principally, by lice. *Pediculus Humanus*—the 'common louse of man'—is a small flat wingless insect, not unlike a button. It has strongly developed claws that it uses for clinging to its unwilling hosts. Probably, such lice have existed for as long as there have been humans to infest— certainly, tiny dry discs that were once the bodies of lice have been found on ancient Egyptian mummies. When present in large numbers, lice can cause intense irritation to the people on whom they are battening. 'Back-scratchers'—small wooden or ivory forks, with long handles—were used by many eighteenth-century ladies who wished to assuage, decorously, the discomforts caused by the lice that were living in their wigs.

Lice, then, were no respecters of persons. Samuel Pepys had noticed with sardonic amusement the prevalence of the 'spotted fever' among the aristocracy. The hungry little creatures throve with particular vigour in dark and badly ventilated dwellings. The tyrannous Window Tax imposed in England in the reign of William and Mary, and made more severe in 1746 and 1747, led to more and more windows being bricked up. This led to a pre-valence of dim and musty rooms, and this, in turn, led to a rapid increase in the ravenous battalions of lice.

The bacillus-carrying vermin came in two distinct varieties—
var Capitis, the head louse, and *var Corporis*, the body louse. Lice of
both these kinds were found in enormous numbers in military
camps during the eighteenth century, and so the movement of
troops tended to spread typhus fever, as well as violence, looting
and rape. Particularly severe outbreaks of the 'putrid fever' were
experienced during the long conflict between Frederick the Great
and Maria Theresa (1740–48) and the Seven Years War (1756–
1763). The French, in the years immediately preceding the Revolution and during the great struggle itself, were notoriously lousy
and typhus-ridden.

Prisons, in the eighteenth century, might have been specially
designed for breeding the causes of fever. They were dark, un-
ventilated, overcrowded places in which human excrement was an
inevitable part of the scene. (How could any more hygienic conditions be expected, when a proportion of the prisoners were
actually chained to iron staples firmly embedded in the walls?)

The prisoners—lacking clean clothes and bedding, and vermin-
ridden—could die of typhus or typhoid fever or any other disease
without seriously troubling society. Unfortunately for society,
though, the prisoners had usually to be tried. Brought from
London's Newgate or some other noisome jail into a court of law,
they carried their lice with them. Inevitably, some at least of the
lice would leave their hosts during the course of a trial and would
crawl off in search of new feeding grounds. 'Black Assizes'—
court sessions followed by disastrous outbreaks of typhus fever—
are recorded on several eventful pages of British legal history.
One of the worst outbreaks of 'jail fever' followed London's Old
Bailey trials of 1750. That metropolitan disaster carried off the
City's Lord Mayor, three stout justices, eight members of the
Middlesex Jury, and more than forty other people who had been
present when the fatal lice set out on their journeys. Each of the
victims of this assault by lice is said to have been sitting on the
left hand side of the court.

Yellow fever—an infective tropical disease, the virus of which is
transmitted by certain species of mosquito—caused more deaths
in the New World than the Old during the eighteenth century.
This dreaded sickness was frequently known as 'vomito negro',
since the sufferer's vomit would often be black with blood, which

signalled internal bleeding, which, in its turn, usually heralded death.

One of the worst epidemics of yellow fever occurred in Philadelphia in 1793. Foremost in fighting the fever in this grim outbreak was the celebrated and energetic Doctor Benjamin Rush. After graduating at Princeton in 1760, Rush had studied at Edinburgh and in the hospitals of London and Paris. In spite of this extended and cosmopolitan training, Doctor Rush's method of treating the fever was conservative—it consisted principally of pouring into the stricken person large quantities of calomel (mercurous chloride, as used for medicinal purposes) and jalap (a purgative root first brought from Xalapa, in Mexico), the dosing being punctuated by the removal of large quantities of blood. (His critics, who were numerous, compared him unkindly but with good reason to Le Sage's Doctor Sangrado.) At the height of the epidemic, the appropriately-named Rush imperilled his own health by treating as many as 150 patients in a single day. He was to die, eventually, of typhus fever in 1813.

Nobody managed to do very much during the eighteenth century to alleviate the distress of those who suffered from the more serious fevers. The work of James Currie—one of the few medical men to try a new therapy in fever cases with any success—was described by the eminent medical historian Silas Weir Mitchell (1829–1914) as having 'absolute genius'. We would not praise Currie quite as wholeheartedly as that today, but we can admire his resilience. He was almost as unsinkable as a cork.

Currie was born at Kirkpatrick Fleming, in Dumfriesshire, Scotland, in 1756. He was the only son of the minister of the church in that small town. When he was a boy he had thoughts, like so many other Scottish lads at that time, of making a career in the practice of medicine. Then he went one day with his father to Glasgow, and there he overheard some men talking about the opportunities offered overseas, to keen youngsters by the rapidly developing colonies. One of the best colonies to emigrate to (said the men) was America, which was directly to the west of Scotland. This conversation fired young Currie with the wish to make his living abroad. His father, surprisingly, sympathized with the boy's ambitions, and the lad landed in Virginia when he was barely fifteen years old. At first, he tried to establish himself as a merchant, but he soon caught one of the endemic fevers and, lowered by its after-effects, was in no fit condition for trade.

Happily, Currie had a relative of his own name—a physician—living at Richmond, Virginia. The older man took the lad into his own home and nursed him back to health. Soon, the younger Currie resolved to give up commerce altogether and he decided to study medicine, instead, as he had originally intended. With the glad confidence of youth, he embarked on a ship bound for Greenock, in Scotland, hoping to graduate at Edinburgh and, later, to return to America to practise.

The young man's plans went wrong, however. Before the ship on which he was travelling had gone far, it was seized by an armed vessel 'in the name of the revolting colonies'. The passengers' luggage was confiscated and young Currie and his fellow voyagers were put ashore on a deserted strip of coast and left to wander.

The War of Independence was then hotting up. Twice, before he could obtain another passage, Currie was conscripted for service in the colonial army. He only managed to escape the draft by making big payments, to 'buy himself out'.

Currie's second attempt to return to Scotland was not much more successful than the first. Again, the ship on which he was travelling was seized. On this second occasion, Currie made a journey of 150 miles in an open boat to appeal against the seizure. He suffered a further attack of fever on this unwanted discursion, and a bad dose of dysentery, and a hurricane added noticeably to his discomforts. After six weeks of these agonizing adventures, Currie and the seized vessel managed to get away. They reached the harbour of St Eustachius in the British West Indies, and there (probably with audible sighs of relief) they dropped anchor.

At St Eustachius, Currie tried to increase his sadly diminished resources by buying goods of various kinds for the British admiral who had been posted to the West Indian Station. He hoped, of course, to make a reasonable profit for himself, but, like all Currie's previous ventures, this enterprise turned out unhappily, for the admiral, taking advantage of a fall in the market, refused to pay for the goods he had asked Currie to purchase. Worn out, frustrated, and practically penniless, Currie caught yet another fever, which was followed by a form of paralysis. He recovered slowly, and was taken on to Antigua, and from there, after a little

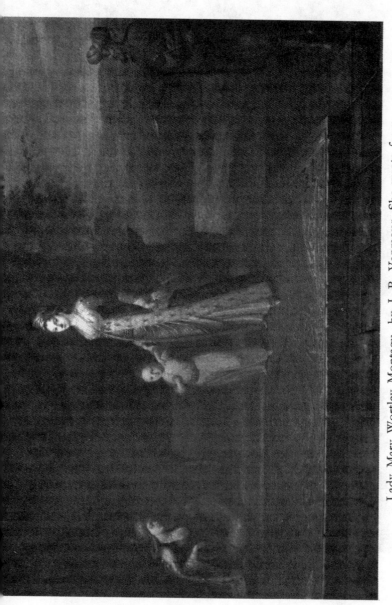

Lady Mary Wortley Montagu, by J. B. Vanmour. She wrote from Turkey in 1717 on the practice of inoculation against smallpox, some sixty years before Dr. Jenner first discovered the safer vaccination used in this country.

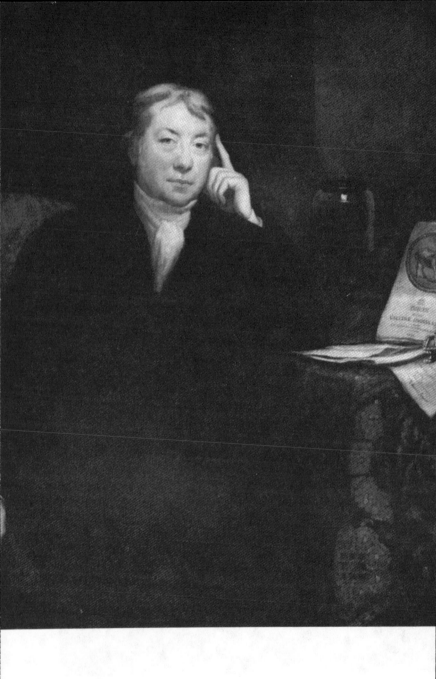

Dr. Edward Jenner of Berkeley, by J. Northcote, 1803.

delay, he sailed for England. Many storms delayed the vessel on which he was travelling and she was twice nearly wrecked, but she struggled into East London's Deptford docking places at last on 2 May 1777.

In the autumn of that year Currie, restored partially to health, started to study medicine at Edinburgh. He had little money to live on, but he was ready to work hard, and the Scottish professors soon noticed that they had an exceptionally gifted and determined student in their midst. But poor Currie seems to have been accident-prone (or, more accurately perhaps, 'fever-prone'). On the first day of the following September he set out for a thirty-two mile walk, for pleasure, with one of his fellow students. Twice, during the day, the young men stopped to bathe and then, after sundown, Currie went into the water for a third time—into the River Tweed, which felt, he remembered afterwards, extra-ordinarily cold. As a result of this indulgence, Currie contracted rheumatic fever—a disorder that almost certainly began the affection of his heart which was repeatedly to interrupt his work, and which led, eventually, to his premature retirement and early death.

Although he had intended to return to America once he had qualified, Currie, very much less healthy than he had been, settled instead in Liverpool—then a growing Merseyside town with extensive moorings—and there, by diligence and by deliberately disregarding his own disabilities he built up a successful practice. Then, in 1797, he published at Liverpool the considerable work by which he earned a tiny niche in medical history, his *Reports on the Effects of Water, cold and warm, as a Remedy in Fever and Febrile Diseases, whether applied to the Surface of the Body or used as a Drink, with Observations on the Nature of Fever and on the Effects of Opium, Alcohol, and Inanition.*

In this book, Currie told how he, himself, being so persistent a sufferer from fevers, had noticed, with the greatest interest, an account given in the *London Medical Journal*, by a Doctor William Wright, formerly resident in the island of Jamaica. Doctor Wright had been on a ship bound for Liverpool from Montego Bay when a hired sailor on board had developed a fever with symptoms of the greatest malignity. The doctor had attended this sailor often, but could not persuade the sick seaman to allow himself to be moved from a dark and confined situation to an airier and more convenient part of the ship. As he had refused medicines, too, and food, the sailor had died on the eighth day of his illness.

By his attention to the sick man, the doctor had himself caught the contagion, and for four days had suffered severe pains and delirium. Then, on the fifth day of his illness, the doctor had observed that when he was taken on deck, his pains were greatly diminished: the colder the air there, he had found, the better he felt. So, he had decided to put into practice on himself a kind of shock treatment that he had often wished to try on others suffering from fevers similar to his own:

> ... September 9th,—Having given the necessary directions, about three in the afternoon, I stripped off all my clothes, and threw a sea-cloak loosely about me till I got upon the deck, when the cloak also was laid aside; three buckets full of salt water were then thrown at once on me; the shock was great but I felt immediate relief. The headach [*sic*] and other pains instantly abated and a fine glow and diaphoresis succeeded. Towards evening, the febrile symptoms threatened a return, and I had again recourse to the same method as before, with the same good effect. I now took food with an appetite, and for the first time had a sound night's rest . . .

On the following day, Doctor Wright had used the cold bath twice. On the day after that, all his unpleasant symptoms had vanished, but he was doused with cold water twice again, to forestall any possibility of a relapse.

Immediately he read this account, Currie had determined to follow his colleague's example, and it was not long before he got an opportunity of putting this resolve into effect.

His chance came in December 1787, when a contagious fever made its appearance in the Liverpool Infirmary. For some time past, the weather had been extremely cold, which, in Currie's words, 'prevented the necessary degree of ventilation', and the infection spread rapidly. Eight of the affected patients were in Currie's care, and on seven of them, for the first time, he used 'the affusion of cold water, in the manner described by Dr Wright'. Of these seven patients, all made a satisfactory recovery.

Currie's book, in which he announced this and further successes, went into four editions. The object of the book was to establish three rules in the treatment of fevers:

(a) In the early stages, the fever should be treated by the pouring of cold water over the patient's body.
(b) In the later stages of the fever, the patient's temperature should be reduced by bathing with tepid water.
(c) In all stages of the fever, the patient should be given large amounts of cold water to drink.

For fifteen hundred years at least, cold bathing had been tried from time to time as a treatment for fevers, but Currie was the first exact observer of its effects, and his were the first medical observations in which readings taken with a clinical thermometer were systematically recorded:

... Jan 1, 1790. A nurse in the fever ward of the Infirmary having several patients under her care, caught the infection. She was seized with violent rigors, chilliness, and wandering pains, succeeded by great heat, thirst and head-ache. Sixteen hours after the first attack, her heat in the axilla [armpit] was 103° of Fah [Fahrenheit], her pulse 112 in the minute and strong, her thirst great, her tongue furred, and her skin dry.

Five gallons of salt water, of the temperature of 44° were poured over her naked body, at five o'clock in the afternoon, and after being hastily dried with towels, she was replaced in bed, when the agitation and sobbing had subsided heat and head-ache were gone, and the thirst nearly gone. Six hours afterwards she was found perfectly free of fever, but a good deal of debility remained ...

After reading Currie's authoritative book, some unsophisticated physicians who could think of no better alternative were persuaded to try cold water applications in the treatment of fevers, and, as doctors today would agree, it is possible that a few lives may have been saved in severe visitations of scarlet fever and the typhoid. Currie's tomb in the parish church at Sidmouth, in Devon, is graced by an epitaph written by a Professor Smyth of

Cambridge. One couplet in this elegant literary exercise commemorates the Liverpool doctor's unorthodox contribution to practical medicine:

> ... Art taught by thee shall o'er the burning frame
> The healing freshness pour and bless thy name ...

Misfortune dogged poor Currie even beyond the grave. Long before more scientific methods of dealing with fevers had become generally available, his name had been largely forgotten.

6

Going to Hospital
in the Eighteenth Century

... There were no water closets. The bread was excellent ...

JOHN HOWARD

Hospitals, in the eighteenth century, were intended for the very poor, not for those who could afford private treatment at home, or in some hired apartment. In many respects, as we shall see, these institutions were quite unlike hospitals as we know them today.

At the beginning of the century, there were only two great general hospitals in London—St Bartholomew's, north of the Thames, and St Thomas's, south of the river.

St Bartholomew's was part of the monastic establishment that had been founded by Rahere—said by some to have been King Henry I's court jester—as far back as the year 1123. In the 577th year of its existence, Rahere's hospital was still little more than a refuge for penniless sick people. This refuge was neither very restful nor very clean, but at least, within its crowded, malodorous and noisy wards, the impoverished could get food, a bed, and physic, all of which would probably have been lacking in their own sparsely-provided homes. St Thomas's—founded by the monks of Southwark more than a century after Rahere started building at Smithfield—was no more advanced or comfortable than the senior Infirmary, but it did, by the standards of the day, equally valuable work.

Paris, at the beginning of the eighteenth century, offered the crumbling Hôtel Dieu as a general place of sanctuary for the sick poor. This venerable institution—almost certainly the oldest hospital in Europe—is supposed to have been founded in the year 660 by St Landry, the Bishop of Paris. By 1700 it was providing homes, of a kind, for numerous families who could afford no other dwelling. These permanently established inmates needed to make a living. So they followed a variety of trades within the hallowed precincts. They slaughtered animals. They removed the dead animals' hides, and tanned them. They used the tallow they obtained from some of the dead animals for making candles, which they sold. All this primitive activity, carried on at such close quarters, can hardly have been good for the health of the genuinely sick patients in the Hôtel Dieu. With nowhere else to go, the genuinely sick patients had to put up with the sounds and the sights and the smells.

They had to put up, too, with the shortage of beds. In the year 1709, when there were at least nine thousand people sleeping each night in the Hôtel Dieu, there were only about a thousand beds there—six hundred large, and four hundred small—to accommodate them. Some of those beds may have contained as many as ten very sick invalids huddled uncomfortably together.

During the eighteenth century, the usefulness of hospitals came to be recognized in most of the civilized countries of the world. By 1800—besides St Bartholomew's and St Thomas's Hospitals mentioned already—the Westminster Hospital (1719), Guy's Hospital (1721), St George's Hospital (1733), the London Hospital (1740) and the Middlesex Hospital (1745) had been built in the British capital, to take one city only, and these great centres of healing and teaching were all functioning busily. (They still survive and function busily today.) A variety of specialist hospitals had been opened in London, too, and a few lying-in hospitals. From that account, it might seem as if no poor sick person in London would ever again need to die neglected and forgotten in some noisome gutter. Alas! This was far from being the case. For, no hospital, even in that age of growing enlightenment, could afford to take in its patients automatically, through a welcoming-everyone, ever-open door. Thomas Guy, in proposing and financing the foundation of his great 'Hospital for Incurables' instructed his executors:

> ... To receive and entertain therein four hundred poor persons, or upwards, labouring under any distempers, infirmities or disorders, thought capable of relief by physic or surgery ...

The executors—later to be the governors of the hospital—spotted an apparent contradiction in terms in this, and they were careful to define exactly and publicly the word 'incurable'. Mr Guy had suspected, they said, that the word, used without any qualification, was of too large and indefinite a signification:

> ... And, indeed, People generally understood by it, such as labour'd under distempers, loss of limbs, blindness, and other natural or accidental deformities, and even age itself. And if taken in such an extensive sense, his Hospital must soon have become an Almshouse, in which (to use his own Words) Parishes, as well as particular persons, would shift off from themselves the burthen of their dependents and indigent relations, to be provided for during their lives ...

Having foreseen this possible misuse of his new hospital, Mr Guy had spoken with great concern on the matter to several of his executors, they reported, and had left to their absolute discretion the question of the admission of the 'several species or kinds of sick persons deemed or called incurables' and also the length of time that they should be accommodated in the hospital. Not having unlimited funds at their disposal, the governors proposed to admit only those 'thought capable of relief by physic or surgery'.

So, potential in-patients had to sue humbly for admission. This is a first-hand account of the conditions that prevailed in Mr Guy's hospital shortly after it opened:

> ... 'Taking-in Day' was Thursday in each week. Having made their petitions, in due form, the applicants, if accepted, proceeded to the Admission Room, male or female. There, they awaited the arrival of the Physician or Surgeon. South, long a surgeon at St Thomas', tells how the physician would make a close enquiry into the history and symptoms of the applicant and would set out the case record in full in Latin, watched and assisted by his pupils if he had any. The surgeon would arrive at his conclusion after only a cursory examination. Whether the examination were short or long, the conclusions arrived at had a surprising sameness—the physicians' cases were most often

admitted as suffering from 'An internal complaint'; the usual surgical label was 'Bad Leg'. Really urgent cases had their cards marked with the physician's of surgeon's initials three times repeated. Intermediate urgency twice repeated. Not really urgent, once. The cards were then taken to a Steward who would assign the patients to such beds as were available, according to their degree of urgency as marked on the cards. A single bed in each ward was always left empty, reserved for any emergency case that might arrive before the next 'Take-In' . . .

In spite of the apparent sameness of the examiners' verdicts, a great variety of cases was taken into Guy's and the other London hospitals during the eighteenth century. In the first month after St George's Hospital was opened, sixty-five patients were admitted for treatment. The list of their ailments can still be studied. It included:

Consumption	10 patients, of whom 2 died
Intermitting Fever	8 patients, of whom 1 died
Diarrhoea	1 patient, of whom 1 died
Rheumatism	5 patients, of whom 1 died
Jaundice	1 patient, cured
Chlorosis	2 patients, 1 cured
Herpes	1 patient, cured
Albugo	1 patient, discharged for 'irregularity'
Fractures	3 patients
Ulcers	11 patients (of whom 3 were 'foul' or suffering from a venereal disease)
Tumours of the Breast	2 patients (1 being cancerous)
Caries of the Leg	2 patients
Glandular Tumours	2 patients

And, one patient with each of these: ringworm, rupture, stone in the bladder, scorbutic eruptions, flux, contusion, gravel, worm fever, pain in breasts, palsy, ophthalmia, fever, asthma, dropsy, spinaventosa and colic.

In one of the lectures he gave to the surgical students at St

Bartholomew's Hospital some time before 1760, the celebrated Doctor Percival Pott mentioned that among the casualty patients admitted to the hospital he had been required to treat a girl who had been tossed by an ox in Smithfield Market; a man who had been thrown from a horse on to the rails there; a man who had been injured by a mob on Tower Hill who were trying to rescue a sailor from a press gang; and a young man who, playing at cudgels in Moorfields, had been stunned by a stroke on the forehead.

While there was a bed for each of the patients admitted during the eighteenth century to the principal London hospitals (except the Bethlehem Hospital, of which more later) the provision of suitable bedding posed certain foreseeable problems. Early in the century, the members of the governing body of St Thomas's Hospital expressed the hope, optimistically, that their patients would bring their own bed linen. By 1754, the governors of the hospital must have seen this, at least in part, as their own responsibility, for when, in that year, they instructed the matron in her duties, they told her that:

> . . . She must take care that no Ruggs, Blankets, Beds [mattresses], Bolsters or Curtains be laid aside as useless till she have well examin'd them and such as by mending may be made fit for further Service she must give orders that they be so mended accordingly . . .

Benjamin Harrison Junior succeeded his father as Treasurer of Guy's Hospital in 1797 at the age of twenty-five. By that time, as we shall see, the hospital was being so badly run that it was almost running down. Keenly, the young man compiled a set of strict rules for the management of the domestic economy:

> . . . All Patients admitted into this Hospital must, before they be received into the Ward, be clean from Vermin and furnished with a Change of Body-Linen, Stockings, Neck-cloth, Stock, or Handkerchief, and to pay to the Sister Two Shillings and Ninepence, for *Two Towels, a Tin Pot, a Knife, a Spoon, an Earthen Plate, and five Pair of Sheets,* and if any Part of the Number of Sheets is not expended during their Continuance,

the Sister shall return Three-pence per Pair; and if any more is used they shall pay Three-pence per Pair; but any Person . . . whose Securities refuse to find them clean Linen &c notwithstanding their being admitted by the Governors, shall be brought to the Steward to be discharged . . .

The patients in the eighteenth-century London hospitals appear to have been reasonably well fed, though the solid food they were offered can hardly be called exciting. A sizeable bequest left to St Bartholomew's Hospital by the wealthy Doctor John Radcliffe enabled the governors to improve considerably the 'dyet for the poore'. On Sundays, before the gift, the patients had received:

10 Ounces of Wheaten Bread
 6 Ounces of Beef boyled without bones
 1 Pint and a half of Beef Broth
 1 Pint of Ale Cawdle at Night
 3 Pints of Seven Shilling Beer

After the gift, the patients were given, each Sunday:

12 Ounces of Wheaten Bread
 8 Ounces of Beef boyled without bones
 1 Pint of Milk Pottage in the Morning
 1 Pint of Ale Cawdle at Night
 3 Pints of Beer
 1 Pint and a half of Beef Broth

Meat was served on three days in each week only, before the bequest arrived, but beer was regarded as an everyday necessity, before and after.

We have little first-hand information about the almost intolerable conditions in which eighteenth-century hospital patients spent their days and nights, but from the rules and regulations issued from time to time by the various boards of governors or their officers, and from the criticisms made by the prison-reformer John Howard after he had made a tour of inspection, we can see that the little band of dedicated elderly women who tried to feed, nurse and generally care for the boisterous inmates had an extremely difficult job. The patients' language, to start with, must have been habitually and compulsively foul:

> . . . The Patients shall not Swear or take Gods Name in Vain nor Revile nor miscall one another, nor strike or beat one another . . .

ordered the governing body of St Thomas's Hospital in 1754. Later in the century, young Benjamin Harrison, at the neighbouring Guy's Hospital, tried to curb the patients' obscenity by threatening explicit penalties:

> . . . If any Patient curse or swear, or use any prophane or Lewd Talking, and it be proved on them by two Witnesses, such Patient shall, for the first Offence, lose their next Day's Diet, and for the second Offence lose two Day's Diet, and the third be discharged . . .

Drunkenness, in the wards, must have presented great and continuing difficulties to the poor women who were responsible for maintaining some kind of order. During most of the eighteenth century, after the foundation of the hospital, the patients at Guy's who were capable of doing so seem to have wandered in and out of the place more or less as they pleased. They attended the hospital for meals and for such medical care as might be provided. The rest of their time, they spent in the ale-houses of the neighbourhood. The patients at St Thomas's were just as free and easy, observed John Howard, adding that there was 'no proper attention to the gates, so that the adjoining gin-shops often prevent the efficacy of medicine and diet'. Benjamin Harrison the Younger—still smarting, evidently under John Howard's censure—cracked down hard on all insobriety:

> . . . If any Patient be found strolling about the Streets, or frequenting Publick-Houses, or Brandy Shops, they forfeit their next Day's Diet . . . If any Patient do privately bring into this Hospital any Spirituous Liquors, such as are not allowed by the Doctors or Surgeons, or fetch such Liquors for any other Patient, both the Patient bringing, and the Patient sending are to be discharged . . .

The young Treasurer of Guy's tried to clean up the hospital, by his regulations, in other respects:

> ... If any Patient be found guilty of any Indecency, or commit any Nuisance in the Squares of the Hospital shall lose their next Day's Diet ...

Economically, he expected the patients to help with the general running of the establishment:

> ... If any Patient that is able neglect or refuse to assist their fellow Patients that are weak, or confined to their Beds, or to assist when called on by the Sister, Nurse or Watch, in cleaning the Ward, helping down with their Stools, fetching Coals, or any other necessary Business relating to their Ward, or shall absent themselves at the Time they know such Business must be done, they shall, for the first Offence, forfeit their next Day's Diet; and for the second Offence, and persisting therein, they shall be discharged by the Steward ...

In 1752 the governors of the two great united London hospitals—St Thomas's and Guy's—ordered that their patients, when going to their meals and beds, should crave God's blessing, and on returning from them should return thanks to God. A proper person should be appointed to read at the desk on Sunday, the governors said, and on Friday mornings that person should read out aloud, in every ward, the rules and orders that were to be obeyed by the patients. Forty-five years later, the virtuous young Treasurer of Guy's was trying, in his turn, to inaugurate a new era of sweetness and light, 'by order of the Governing Body':

> ... On Sunday Evening, between the Hours of Six and Eight in the Winter and Seven and Nine in the Summer, some sober Person in each Ward, appointed by the Sister, shall, at the Desk, with an audible Voice, Distinctly read two Chapters, one in the Old Testament and one in the New (and every Evening some Person shall, at the Desk, read the Prayers appointed, and all Patients that are able shall attend at the Desk, and behave

with Decency and Devotion) on Sunday. Likewise, at the same Time read a Section of the Duty of Man, or the Practice of Piety. To all which religious Observations, every Patient shall attend with decent Behaviour; but if any Person shall be observed to mock or scoff at these or any other religious Directions, such Persons shall be immediately discharged ...

What were they really like, these sisters and their helpers, who had to look out for smuggled spirituous liquors and to appoint proper persons to read aloud from the Scriptures? Since Charles Dickens created the immortal Sairey Gamp, the idea has been widely accepted that all pre-Florence Nightingale nurses were criminally uncouth. Towards the end of the eighteenth century, it has to be admitted, the nursing staff at Guy's and other hospitals had come to be recruited from 'a very inferior type of person'—Benjamin Harrison the Younger had to recognize that fact when he was appointed to his Treasurership—but no one, reading through the minutes of the hospitals' governors during the greater part of the period under review, could fail to be impressed by the infrequency of the complaints made against the members of those hospitals' staffs. Those who fell from grace were all the more noticeable for their rarity.

There were the Sister and Nurse of Mary's Ward in St Bartholomew's Hospital, for instance, who, on 7 November 1708, were reprimanded for 'not being so tender as they ought to be to ye poor patients under their care ... '

Two years later, Ann Keble and Ann Cesar who had been patients in the same great old London hospital complained to the governors that:

... Sarah Owen Sister to Cathrines [St Catherine's] ward doth demand and take of every patient sent into that ward 2s 6d and causeth them to spend 6d: That Ann Deane her Helper likewise demands a Shilling of each patient and that the said Sister washeth her Sons and daughters linnen and makes the patients Iron the same. Upon examining of Ann Preston, Martha Gold, Phillis Chamlett and Mary Browning now patients in that ward concerning the same Complaint they all declared that the said Sister and Helper do make such demands and that some patients have pawned their Cloths to raise money to satisfye them otherwise they are neglected and slighted. And that the same Sister doth cause her Sons and daughters linnen to be Iron'd by the patients . . .

It was 'thereupon thought fitt and Ordered', by the governors, that the said Sister and Helper should be discharged.

One of the beadles at St Bartholomew's Hospital—a Robert Cracraft—was a constant cause of concern to the governing body. Having been previously 'repremanded for abusing of his Neighbour' and told that if he continued to be troublesome he should be 'forthwith dismist', he was in really hot water on 9 May 1709, when the sister of the cutting [operating] ward reported him for refusing to call a surgeon to a patient who had been lately operated on for the stone in the bladder and whose wound was bleeding. Cracraft was 'discharged of his place till further order'. He was reinstated, on 'praying to be restored to his former office, and promising for the future to behave himself'. Re-engaged at the same time was Cracraft's fellow beadle, Thomas Trigg, who had been sacked for being drunk while on duty.

Nine months later, Cracraft was up before the board again, in spite of his vows. On this occasion, John Middleton, the porter to the hospital had complained that the beadle:

. . . Was very remiss and negligent in performing of his duty and in watching and being in the Cloyster of this Hospital when it is his turn and particularly on Tuesday last upon telling him thereof the said Cracraft did abuse the said Porter by giving him the lye and calling him saucy rascall and using other approbious language the which he could not deny . . .

The governors ordered, this time, that Cracraft should be suspended from his duties for a month, and for so long after that as the board should think fit.

A more serious complaint was considered by the governors of St Bartholomew's in 1717. It was made by the widow of a man who had recently died while he was a patient in the hospital. According to this sad woman, her husband's body, after being interred in the burial place at Moorfields, had been

... Taken up by ye Grave Digger and Sold to some Surgeons which Corps was stopped at an Inn in a hamper to be sent to Oxford and informed the Board that the Grave Digger hath been committed to Newgate for that fact and the Surgeons bound over to answer the same at the Sessions ...

The widow, being poor, asked that the governors of the hospital should give orders for the prosecution of the said gravedigger and the surgeons. She asked, too, that the board should foot the bill for all the legal charges that would be involved. The governors agreed to do as the widow requested and ordered their clerk to pursue the matter with the utmost rigour.

The words quoted at the beginning of this chapter, ' ... There were *no water closets*. The bread was *excellent* ... ' were written by the great reformer John Howard shortly after he had visited St Thomas's Hospital in Southwark, and they indicate one of the least savoury features of eighteenth-century hospital life. Indoor sanitation was, at most hospitals at that time, a remote dream of the future, like the aeroplane.

If the St Bartholomew's Hospital governors' records are to be believed, no patient during the whole of the eighteenth century complained about the sanitary arrangements of the hospital. This is quite surprising, for during the greater part of the century the place was cleared of human excrement in much the same way as a farmyard of the period might have been cleared—the droppings and outpourings of the patients and staff were carried in pails and buckets to a large open cesspool situated just outside one of the main wards. From this nauseating pond, the solid matter would be regularly removed, in bulk, and would be carried away by a 'nightsoil carrier'.

The crudity of this system does not appear to have worried the hospital authorities overmuch. In 1729 they invited James Gibbs to design a fine new building for them. Architecturally, the Gibbs block at St Bartholomew's is superb. It has a magnificent Assembly Room, for the use of the members of the board and their guests, and this great room, with its polished wood floor, has one of the finest plasterwork ceilings to be found in any comparable meeting place of the period in the whole of the world. It has a grand staircase, lit by an immense chandelier, up and down which the governors of the hospital would walk in solemn procession, holding their specially painted wands of office. On the walls to right and left of this grand staircase, William Hogarth, Britain's most famous artist, having been elected a member of the governing body, painted two of his most impressive mural decorations— *The Pool of Bethesda*, in which the sick are shown being restored to health by their Blessed Lord, and *The Good Samaritan*, with its obvious references to healing. Magnificent the new Gibbs building at St Bartholomew's may have been, but the wards in that building were not served by one single hygienic lavatory. Every morning, the buckets and pails had to be carried down one of the not-so-grand back staircases and emptied into the foul seething pit about which nobody in the hospital wanted to know, but which nobody in the hospital could ever forget.

Guy's was one of the first public hospitals to take seriously the problem of sanitation. In 1774 a 'beautiful new Common Privy' was constructed there. From this privy a great sewer 'was carried through the First Square and across St Thomas's Street in order to remove the nauseous smells which continually arose from the construction of the old Privy'. John Howard, visiting Guy's fourteen years after that, admired the water closets in the new wards which worked in an ingenious way, being [he reported]:

... Constantly supplied with fresh water, from a reservoir; they empty and fill the basin by opening the door. They are so simply constructed that they require little attention, and are not liable to be easily put out of repair. They are free from ill scents. The basin is of earthen or queen's ware, glazed; and it is always charged with water, being supplied afresh every time the patient leaves the closet. The door acts on the cistern by a common lever, and the same operation discharges all that is left in the basin ...

By the time Benjamin Harrison the Younger assumed the Treasurership of the hospital, the flushing mechanisms in the privies were permanently out of order, and the basins were 'cracked and offensive'.

The discomforts caused to eighteenth-century patients by a hospital's 'nauseous smells' were bad enough. Worse, even, than these were the irritations caused by the lice that infested the wards. The records of St Bartholomew's Hospital for 1712 contain this entry:

... James Jones Joiner did agree to clear the severall Wards within this Hospitl of Buggs for five Guineys to be paid him immediately [and] eight pounds at ye years end ...

In 1735 the Court of Committees at Guy's Hospital ordered that twenty pounds should be paid to one John Hilberdine 'on account of his services in killing buggs'. Four years later, the members of the court were told that the patients in the hospital were 'annoyed in a very grevious manner with Buggs'. They left it to a Mr Troar to take such steps as he should think most effective for clearing the mens' wards of the annoying little creatures. The lice continued to thrive.

In 1765 Samuel Sharp, the first surgeon appointed permanently to the staff of Guy's Hospital, became seriously ill from overwork. When he had recovered sufficiently to be able to travel, he set off on a tour of Italy. In his *Letters from Italy*, published in the following year, Sharp reported that he had noticed in the hospital at Florence a bedstead with an iron frame:

... In the hospitals at London [he continued], bugs are frequently a greater evil to the patient than the malady for which he seeks an hospital; and could I have interest enough with the Governors to bring about an imitation of this frame, I should be exceedingly rejoiced in the comfort it will afford to so many thousands of miserable wretches that are tormented, sometimes even to death, by these nauseous vermin ...

Twenty-two years later, John Howard found that some of the new wards at Guy's had 'iron bedsteads and hairbeds' and were clean and fresh. In several of the old wards, he found, the beds and testers were made of wood, and were still infested with lice. As the chief bug-catcher to the hospital was being paid, at this time, as much as any of the physicians and surgeons, the introduction of the expensive iron bedsteads was expected to prove, in the long run, an economy.

During the greater part of the eighteenth century, the teaching lectures given at the principal London hospitals were designed to make and educate surgeons. 'Medicine was but little taught, and that little was intended for the general practitioner—then called "apothecary"—whose studies at a school needed not, at that time, to extend beyond six or twelve months,' asserted Professor Quain, in a lecture he gave at University College, London, in 1874. 'English students habitually went to Paris to study medicine, where the courses were complete and supported by government.'

Joseph Warner, who was a surgeon at Guy's Hospital from 1745 to 1790, was a student there as early as 1734. He recalled, towards the end of his life, that when he had first become acquainted with St Thomas's Hospital and Guy's Hospital, the rules of both establishments had laid down that each surgeon was allowed to receive four pupils and four dressers at a time, inclusive of apprentices. All the money received from the apprentices and dressers became the whole and sole property of the surgeon or surgeons with whom such apprentices and dressers were entered at the steward's office of the respective hospitals. The pupil's business was only to look on, he said, 'and to make such an enquiry as he should chuse of the surgeon who was then attending.'

William Hunter, whose own lectures were to widen medical and anatomical knowledge so extensively, used to make, in his introductory talks, some scathing remarks about the way in which he himself had been taught:

... I attended, as diligently as the generality of students do, one of the most reputable courses of anatomy in Europe. There I learned a good deal by my ears, but almost nothing by my eyes; and therefore hardly anything to the purpose. The defect was that the professor was obliged to demonstrate all the parts of the body, except the bones, nerves, and vessels, upon one dead body.

There was a foetus for the nerves and blood-vessels; and the operations of surgery were explained, to very little purpose indeed, upon a dog. And in the whole course which I attended in London, which was by far the most reputable that was given here, the professor used only two dead bodies in his course.

The consequence was, that at one of these places all was harangue,—very little was distinctly seen; in the other the course was contracted into too small a compass of time, and therefore several material points were left out altogether . . .

Travelling round Europe in a prolonged tour of inspection of the continent's principal hospitals, prisons and lazarettos, John Howard was able to compare the establishments he visited abroad with those he looked at in London and, in a few instances, the English hospitals came off badly. He admired the way the patients' beds were set in spacious recesses at Toledo and Burgos. (At the Westminster Hospital, the old beds were 'crowded against the walls'.) He approved of the curtains supplied for privacy at Genoa and Savona. In some Swedish hospitals, he observed:

> . . . A very good mode of sweetening the beds: on every fine day a certain number were brought into the open air, and beaten and brushed on a deal machine made for that purpose. I could wish that such a practice were adopted in our hospitals, and that the rest of the bedding were more frequently washed and aired . . .

But the Swedes were, as so often since, exceptional and ahead of their time. Conditions in the Hôtel Dieu, in Paris, were so abominable, in 1788, that the attendants could not bear to enter the wards in the mornings unless they held to their faces sponges dipped in vinegar.

What chances of success, in those circumstances, had the surgeons?

7

The Shadow of the Knife

... My shroud of white, stuck all with yew,
O! Prepare it ...

WILLIAM SHAKESPEARE, 1564–1616

Compared with the numerous and varied operations that are performed in hospitals today, the operations attempted by surgeons in the eighteenth century were severely limited in range. This apparent lack of enterprise was not entirely due to the surgeons being deficient in technical skill.

The surgeons' scope was limited more drastically by their inability to prevent the unpleasant and frequently fatal consequences of cutting, in unclean air and surroundings, into human flesh. As we have seen, septic fevers and other infections were prevalent in all hospitals—they were found even in Swedish hospitals—and as the surgeons knew that if they cut deeply, the after-effects would be virtually certain to kill their patients, they did not rush to use the knife except for the ubiquitous practice of 'bleeding'. Of necessity, they ventured to remove easily accessible cancers of the skin, breast and the subcutaneous tissues because they knew, from previous experience, that post-operative infection on the surface of the body was unpleasant, but was not necessarily lethal. They rarely, if ever, performed operations on organs that were deep in the abdominal cavity because they knew —also empirically—that any interference of this kind would lead almost inevitably to peritonitis, and they knew, too, that peritonitis would lead almost inevitably to death.

One of the most enterprising of all eighteenth-century surgeons was Lorenz Heister, who became Professor of Surgery and Anatomy at Altdorf, in Germany. In his youth, Heister used to spend a lot of his time at the great popular fairs at which travelling 'operators' could be seen plying their trade. These wandering surgeons used to undertake, in a rough and ready way, operations that more permanently situated practitioners did not dare to perform. In the year 1700, when he was a lad of seventeen, Heister visited the fair at Frankfurt:

> ... It is usual for a number of oculists, and other operators, to resort to Frankfort at the fair time, to undertake the cure of persons afflicted with ruptures, cataracts, the stone, excrescences, hare-lips, and such like disorders; there being, at the time I am speaking of, no physician or surgeon at Frankfort who cared to perform these operations ...

At Amsterdam, Heister saw for the first time the operation for the remedying of a hare-lip being carried out. The operation was performed on a child of two by Mr Van Bortel, an eminent surgeon of the city. Heister noted carefully Mr Van Bortel's methods:

> ... He ordered one of his assistants to seat himself on a chair, and take the child on his lap, holding it fast round the waist, at the same time confining the child's hands. Another assistant stood behind, holding his head on both sides to keep it steady. A third held the child's right leg, and a fourth the left, whereby he was fixed immoveable. Then taking a good pair of scissors in his right hand, and with the index-finger and thumb of the left, taking hold of one edge of the fissure, he cut off about as much as the breadth of the back of a knife, and the same he immediately did on the other edge; then wiping off the blood from the mouth and lip with a sponge, and having three proper needles ready, he passed the first through both lips of the fissure, about the breadth of the back of the knife from the edge of the wound, the second in the middle, and the third at the bottom, and fixing a double thread to the uppermost, he twisted it backwards and forwards several times, and in the same manner to the two other needles; after rubbing the wound with a little honey of roses, he applied a narrow bandage from the part to the back of the head, bringing it round to the forehead, where he tied it, and pinned it fast to the child's cap behind, and on each side. The fifth day the middle needle

was removed; the sixth day the uppermost, and on the seventh the other; after anointing the part with vulnerary balsam, he applied a narrow strip of plaster to the part, upon the falling off of which, the wound was perfectly healed . . .

Heister taught that only a few instruments should be used for surgery and he recommended, too, that they should be simple. ('Great apparatus,' he said, 'having been invented more for the sake of pomp than real utility.') He made exceptions in the case of the instruments needed for such special operations as lithotomy—cutting, to remove a stone or stones from the bladder— and trepanation (cutting away a portion of the cranium to relieve pressure on the brain). His fancy was caught by a cunningly contrived lancet that could be used for removing the tonsils from unwilling patients without the unwilling patients knowing that their tonsils were being removed:

> . . . I know well [he wrote] that suppurated tonsils may be opened with a lancet or sharp knife; yet for the sake of children and the more delicate and timorous, particularly of the fair sex, we ought to contrive a milder method, as these frequently and obstinately oppose cutting or puncturing with instruments, preferring to be suffocated than suffer themselves to be touched. In which case I think it in no wise repugnant to the wisdom, duty, and conscience of a physician to use deceit in order to save the life of his patient, and to free him quickly from his pain. An instrument maker at Amsterdam showed me a new instrument for opening suppurated tonsils, the inventor of which is unknown to me, with which we may practise an honest deceit upon such a patient. For after the surgeon has introduced into the mouth this instrument (which appears like a spatula and in which is contained the lancet) to depress the tongue to look at the throat, he may push forward the lancet with the thumb, and open the tumour and the patient hardly know anything of the matter . . .

A stone in the bladder can cause excruciating discomfort. Agonies of this kind seem to have been fairly common prior to, and during, the eighteenth century—the unsatisfactory food 'enjoyed' by all but the very wealthy is believed to have contributed appreciably to this state of affairs.

Lithotomy—the operation by which an offending stone is removed from a bladder—was, as the eighteenth century dawned, an exceptionally severe one, and most sufferers from the stone would only agree to be 'cut' if the pain that was tormenting them was making life practically unbearable. Their reluctance to submit, in all-too-painful consciousness, to the knife is easily understood, since the stone-removing operation that was usually performed lasted, under normal circumstances, for nearly an hour and, if the surgeon concerned did not happen to be a virtuoso, could drag on considerably longer.

In this ghastly operation, a huge incision would be made in or near the patient's groin. Using this raw and bleeding aperture as a means of access to the patient's interior mechanisms, the surgeon would proceed to dilate, with specially contrived instruments, the neck of the patient's bladder. Then he, the surgeon, would take a pair of forceps, and with this dangerous implement he would attempt to find, in the sombre recesses of the agonized patient, the offending stone or stones. If he, the surgeon, were exceptionally skilful, or exceptionally lucky and if his gropings went unusually well, the unwanted lumps of calcium carbonate would be detected, and would be withdrawn as quickly as possible from their all-too-sensitive resting places—if necessary, by force. The whole process, in the absence of anaesthetics, must have been an excruciating experience for the surgeon and his assistants, if they had any human feelings at all: it must have been painful beyond belief for the patient.

The physical conditions under which this hazardous operation might be performed were, obviously, important. In August 1709 the governors of St Bartholomew's Hospital

> . . . Ordered that the brick peer in the Cutting Ward be taken away and a convenient light made for the benefitt of cutting patients afflicted with the Stone in the bladder and Mr Strode is desired to give direccons for the doing thereof . . .

Five years later, the governors of the same grand old hospital were keen to see some tangible results. At a meeting held in June 1714, they ordered:

> . . . That the Stones taken out of the Patients Bladders that are cut within this Hospitl be brought into the Compting house [Counting House] and showed to the Treasurer and Govrs. at their next meeting after the said Patients are cutt and hung up in the said Compting house according to ancient Custom . . .

The right to perform on any human being an operation so painful and so dangerous was, correctly, jealously guarded. Throughout the whole of the rest of the eighteenth century, after the foundation of Guy's Hospital, the special permission of the governors had to be obtained before any surgeon might 'cut for the stone'. Mr Hasell Cradock, appointed surgeon to Guy's in 1732, was granted the necessary licence a few months later:

> . . . If a convenient place can be provided for cutting [recorded the governors' clerk], and a ward proper for the cut patients, then Mr Cradock be allowed to cut the next season: and Mr Treasurer is desired to consider of such place and ward . . .

An untold amount of human suffering was spared by a bit of careful thinking done by William Cheselden. Cheselden, born in the year 1688, became a principal surgeon at St Thomas's Hospital in the year 1719. In 1723 he published a *Treatise on the High Operation for the Stone*, in which he described a new approach that could be used for the primary incisions. In spite of Cheselden's tributes to the work done in the field by several of his predecessors, his book was violently attacked in an anonymous pamphlet that is believed to have been written by John Douglas, a rival surgeon and anatomist, who accused Cheselden of being a plagiarist. Not much damage was done to Cheselden's growing reputation by this wild libel, for, shortly after, Cheselden entirely discarded this method of operating, adopting, instead, the so-called 'lateral operation', which was indisputably his own invention, and which enabled him to execute a lithotomy operation, with unparalleled skill and brilliance, in approximately one minute. Frequently, he did the job in less than sixty seconds. His daring innovation reduced the mortality rate in those operated on for the stone from about fifty per cent to under ten per cent, and this impressive success ratio was not improved on until the nineteenth century was nearly over, when an operation known as 'lithotrity'—or, crushing the stone—became fashionable. Cheselden recorded, for posterity, his own views on his remarkable surgical feat:

... What success I had in my private practice I have kept no account of because I had no intention to publish it, that not being sufficiently witnessed. Publicly in St Thomas' Hospital I have cut two hundred and thirteen; of the first fifty, only three died; of the second fifty, three; of the third fifty, eight; and of the last sixty-three, six. Several of these patients had the smallpox during their cure some of which died, but I think not more in proportion than what usually die of that distemper; these are not reckoned among those who died of the operation. The reason why so few died in the first two fifties was that at that time, very few bad cases offered; in the third, the operation being in high request even the most aged and the most miserable cases expected to be saved by it. One of the three that died out of the one hundred and five was very ill with whooping-cough; another bled to death by an artery into the bladder, it being very hot weather at that time. But this accident taught me afterwards, whenever a vessel bled that I could not find, to dilate the wound with a knife till I could see it.

If I have any reputation in this way I have earned it dearly, for no one ever endured more anxiety and sickness before an operation, yet from the time I began to operate all uneasiness ceased and if I have had better success than some others I do not impute it to more knowledge but to the happiness of mind that was never ruffled or disconcerted and a hand that never trembled during any operation ...

In 1719 a young French surgeon named Morand was sent over to England to report upon Mr Cheselden's method of operating for the stone. When he returned to his native country, Morand spoke so highly of the new technique that it soon became known and practised throughout Europe and America.

When serious accidents caused nearly fatal accidents in the eighteenth century, operations had frequently to be performed regardless of their small chances of success. Descriptions of emergency operations of various types are contained in the case book of Richard Austin, who was a pupil at St Thomas's Hospital in January 1726. The book is still carefully preserved in the buildings, near Westminster Bridge, that are at present occupied by St Thomas's.

The patient, in one case, was a man whose gun had burst when he fired it, lacerating his hand very badly. When this man was taken to the hospital, two days after the accident, he was placed in the care of Mr Paul, who was one of the hospital's surgeons. As the patient's hand was black, and obviously mortifying, Mr Paul decided that it ought to be amputated at once.

So, the necessary instruments and dressings were taken from the surgery, into the cutting ward. Richard Austin dutifully listed them:

A tourniquet and tape

A knife, a 'catlin' [a long narrow double-edged sharp pointed straight knife used for amputating] and a saw

Forceps and ligatures

An armed needle

A sponge and 'sissars'

Lint and buttons

A large armed 'pledget' [a soft compress of lint, or some other absorbent material], a dry one, a long cloth, a cross cloth, and a double roller

Word had been passed round the hospital that there was to be an operation, and the pupils came trooping in to see it. As Mr Cheselden happened to be on the premises, and as he happened to be the principal surgeon to the hospital at that time, he too came into the ward—ostensibly, in the rôle of a spectator.

First, the patient was placed in a good light. Then, Mr Paul's apprentice fixed the tourniquet in position on the man's arm and twisted it tightly. While he was doing this, Mr Paul tied a piece of tape round the lower end of the man's forearm, to act as a guide for his knife. Mr Cheselden—interfering, one might say—suggested that before Mr Paul did this, he should have pulled up the patient's skin. (The 'flap' operation, which made some provision for covering the ends of a patient's bones, was already known and was being practised at this time.) Mr Paul, not liking his forgetfulness to be noticed and pointed out before so many critical eyes, remarked coolly that he had intended to do that later.

Next, Mr Paul made a circular cut round the whole of the patient's forearm, taking the cut right down to the bones. At this stage, he tried to take Mr Cheselden's advice, by drawing back the soft parts to form a flap, but he found that the tightness of the tourniquet prevented him from doing this. Meanwhile, his assistant was dividing the structures between the two bones with the catlin. The patient, by this time, was shrieking and struggling, for he had been suffering terrible pain during the two days that had elapsed before he was taken to the hospital, and he was not really in a fit state, Robert Austin observed, to face so agonizing an operation with a proper degree of fortitude.

The cutting of the bones came next. First, Mr Paul cut a notch in the radius bone, using his saw. Then, he cut through the ulna bone. He finished by sawing all the way through the radius.

Two arteries, by this time, were spurting blood, and Mr Paul and his assistant picked them up with the armed needle so that they could be ligatured. '*Three* arteries will need a ligature,' observed Mr Cheselden, unable, once again, to resist the temptation to interfere. In accordance with the senior man's advice, the tourniquet was eased. After that had been done, a third artery— the *anterior interosseus*—started to bleed and was successfully picked up and tied.

The raw stump was dressed next, but here Richard Austin's case book becomes confused and difficult to follow—possibly because he was more than a little disturbed by the mounting excitements of the operation. The procedure, however, seems to have followed approximately these stages. First, the exposed ends of the bones were covered with lint, but not before the buttons were dipped in some warm fluid and placed over the ends of the severed arteries. Then, the armed pledget was dipped in something not specified, but possibly water, that was also warm, and the damp dressing was wrapped over the end of the stump. The dry pledget was placed over that. Finally, the cross cloth and the bandage were tied over the preliminary dressings.

Richard Austin's notes do not tell us whether the roller mentioned in the inventory of instruments and dressings was used on this patient or not, but as Mr Cheselden appears to have been in an interfering mood, it probably was. The senior man invariably relied on this implement for keeping the patient's muscles still while he was operating and for keeping the 'softer parts' from shrinking away from the bones. Austin did record the final stages of the amputation, though:

> ... Then the patient was carried to bed and had a *haustus quietans* [soporific draught] and all things tended [tending?] to his ease and quiet, for no man ever endured the operation worse ...

The poor man's stump was dressed every other day after that, with dry dressing 'in ye middle and grey to ye edges to cicatrize'. Fifteen days after the operation, all the ligatures had been cast off. By 10 February 1726—nearly four weeks after the removal of the hand—there were unwelcome developments:

> ... There seem'd as if the bone ends would exfoliate [cast off their outer surfaces, in the form of putrid 'leaves' or scales] because they appeared black and were not covered over as usuall ...

Young Austin was unable to finish the history of the case: 'Opportunity being awanting I saw not ye consequences ... ' But we may safely wager that 'ye consequences', for that poor man who pressed the trigger of his gun with such misplaced confidence, were tragic.

The surgeons who operated in the great London hospitals at the end of the eighteenth century do not seem to have been much more competent than Mr Paul who forgot, while the century was still young, to make his flap.

There was a Mr William Lucas, for instance, who was elected

to the post of surgeon at Guy's Hospital in 1773 and who continued to cut away there until he retired in 1799. For a first-hand view of Mr Lucas, we can turn to the writings of Sir Astley Cooper, one of the greatest surgeons ever to work at Guy's. Sir Astley passed this verdict on Mr Lucas:

> . . . Mr Lucas was a clever manipulator and a neat surgeon, but not an anatomist. He got £300 per annum by bleeding, visited a hundred families, but, he told me, never got more than £500 per annum . . .

Sir Astley could afford to be financially condescending. For many years, his own annual income was more than £15,000—in those days, a very great sum. One incapacitated tycoon is said to have handed Sir Astley a cheque for one thousand guineas, in his nightcap, after Sir Astley performed on him a successful operation for the removal of a stone.

William Lucas's son, William Lucas Junior, succeeded to his father's post in 1799. Sir Astley said of the younger Lucas:

> . . . He had ill-health and could not study anatomy. He was neat-handed, but rash in the extreme, cutting among most important parts as if they were only skin, and making us all shudder from the apprehension of his opening arteries or some other error . . .

Another Guy's official who saw William Lucas Junior at work said of him:

> . . . He was commonly known as Billy. His father had been surgeon at Guy's before him, and had been spoken of as a very excellent surgeon and operator; but the present son was in every respect a very different man. He was tall, ungainly, and awkward; with stooping shoulders, shuffling walk, and as deaf as a post; not overwhelmed with brains of any kind, but very good-natured and easy, and liked by every one. His surgical acquirements were very small, and his operations were badly performed and accompanied with much bungling, if not

worse. He was a poor anatomist and not very good diagnoser, which now and then led him into rather ugly scrapes. There was a story current that Billy, having to amputate the leg, performed the circular operation and made the covering for the bone at the wrong end, the stump being left uncovered and projecting . . .

A Mr William Cooper, who was an uncle of the great Sir Astley, was a surgeon at Guy's from 1783 to 1800. He was 'lively, well-informed and talented'—according to Mr Bransby Cooper, a nephew—but Sir Astley, who became an articled pupil of his father's brother in 1784, said of him:

> . . . My uncle was a man of great feeling—too much so to be a surgeon. He was going to amputate a man's leg in the theatre of the hospital, when the poor fellow, terrified at the array of instruments and appliances, suddenly jumped off the table and bolted off; seeing which, the operator, instead of following the man, and attempting to persuade him to submit to the evil which circumstances rendered necessary, turned round and said, apparently much relieved by his departure, 'By God! I'm glad he's gone' . . .

It is possible to visit, today, an operating theatre that has actually survived from the bad old times before anaesthetics and antiseptic surgery were developed, and a grim place it is, too. The theatre is situated in Southwark, quite near the southern end of London Bridge. It was built in the roof space above St Thomas's Church, and parts of its raised lantern light can be seen if a close study is made of early nineteenth-century engravings of the church and its immediate surroundings. In 1870, a railway company took over the adjoining premises, and the staircase by which the surgeons, staff and students of Old St Thomas's Hospital reached the theatre was bricked up. The theatre, entirely forgotten, was accidentally re-discovered in 1950, when the old church was being adapted for use as the Chapter House for Southwark Cathedral, which is just a stone's throw away on the west side of the Borough High Street.

A visit to the old operating theatre—now, carefully restored, with generous financial help from the Wolfson Foundation—is a chilling experience. The theatre is approached from a subdued entrance in St Thomas's Street, by means of a steep spiral staircase enclosed in cold concave stone walls. Once he, or she, is safely up in the murky roof space over the old church, the visitor can see some well-chosen exhibits. There is a selection of medicinal herbs, for instance, of the kinds that would have been dried there, under the hot, sloping, tiled roof surfaces, in sufficient quantities to satisfy the needs of the two great hospitals, St Thomas's and Guy's, which sprawled over the streets around.

From this interesting attic, the visitor can move into the bleak side room that served, once upon a time, as the ante-chamber to the operating theatre itself. In this small space, after the merciful qualities of anaesthetics had been discovered, patients were wafted, with ether or with chloroform, into unconsciousness.

In the period with which we are dealing, patients taken into that ante-chamber had no such happy relief. They would be given gin, or rum, or some soporific drug, to make their ordeal just a little less harrowing. Then, they would be exhorted to be brave, to be determined and upright, and to clench their hands, while unspeakable things were done to them.

A contemporary illustration, now framed and hanging on the walls, shows what happened to a strong young man who had been exhorted to be brave, to be 'determined and upright', and to clench his hands, once he was guided out through the harmless-looking double doors that are still there, into the operating theatre, which is still there too. The print, in two parts, shows in the first part an operating team about to amputate at the shoulder the young man's shattered arm. The patient is portrayed by the artist as being creditably determined and upright. In the second part, which shows the operation in progress, the young man is seen in a state of complete collapse.

The word 'theatre' is a very appropriate one to apply to the long-lost operating room at Old St Thomas's, for steeply banked standings for spectators are the principal furnishings of the horseshoe-shaped 'auditorium'. A large notice headed REGULATIONS FOR THE THEATRE, on the wall that directly faces the standings, tells how the 'stage' and standings were to be occupied:

> Apprentices and the Dressers of the Surgeon who operates are to stand round the Table. The dressers of the other Surgeons are to occupy the Front Rows. The Surgeon's pupils are to take their Places in the rows above.
> Visitors are admitted by permission of the Surgeon . . .

The walls of the theatre, its furnishings, and the high wooden planked surfaces that fence in the operating arena are painted in dull ochres and duns. These colours were chosen so that they would be as near as possible to the original tones. (The idea that an operating theatre should be mainly white is, of course, relatively modern. No one thought there was any need for special cleanliness until after Joseph Lister had discovered the importance of aseptic conditions during surgery.)

The operating arena, on which the attention of the spectators so closely packed in the standings would be concentrated, is approximately eighteen feet long and ten feet wide. The floor boards of this arena form, in fact, a false floor, being laid on joists which rest upon the true floor. Between these two surfaces there is a five-inch space. Today, this space is empty. In the days when the operating theatre was in regular use, it would have been packed with sawdust. The sawdust would have been necessary for soaking up the blood that ran so copiously off the operating table and down the cracks between the boards. Crimson stains appearing suddenly on the ceiling of the church below might have been embarrassing.

Centrally placed in the arena is the operating table. This is an ordinary kitchen table of a type that might have been made by a village carpenter, and it is not fitted with any accessories except a movable wooden rest for the patient's head. The unpainted, unvarnished and unpolished surfaces of the wooden table are marked, now, with suggestive cuts and crevices. These blemishes must have been made, in the table's heyday, by the saws and hatchets of the less accurate surgeons who did their carving on it. Their deep recesses would have harboured enough germs to wipe out several regiments.

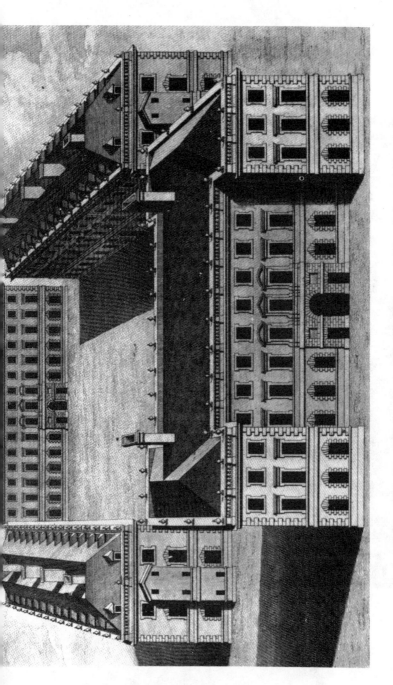

James Gibbs's perspective view of St. Bartholomew's Hospital *c.* 1710.

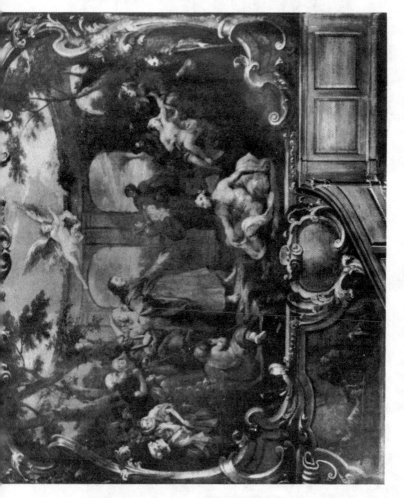

Hogarth's *Pool of Bethesda*, painted on the wall of the Great Hall of St. Bartholomew's Hospital in 1735–6. Many of the prevalent diseases

On the floor beneath the operating table, there is a shallow lidless box or tray. This receptacle was, and is, filled with sawdust. It had a macabre function—it could be kicked, by the surgeon, to any place where it might be especially needed for catching any streams of blood that might run, with particular persistence, over the edge of the operating surface. When the sawdust became so thoroughly impregnated with blood that it was unable to absorb any more, the surgeon would shout out 'More sawdust!' and a fresh box would be placed under the table.

The other furnishings of the old operating theatre have a quaint, domesticated and slightly shabby look about them. They might have been thrown out of the servants' quarters of a depressed country house. There is a large unpainted wooden cupboard, used for the storage of surgical instruments. There is a wooden stand, fitted with a wash-basin that is little larger than a soup plate. Near this, there is a row of pegs on which the surgeons would hang their 'operating coats'—discarded frock coats, usually, which, after they had been used in the theatre for any length of time, would be stiff with dried pus and blood. On entering the theatre to operate, an eighteenth-century surgeon would take off his street coat and then would put on his 'operating coat', rolling up his sleeves and turning up the collar over his white linen to save it from becoming unnecessarily stained. Only the most advanced surgeons, towards the end of the century, ventured to don specially contrived bib-and-apron garments of the type worn chiefly, in later decades, by grocers.

It is difficult for us to appreciate fully, now, how a patient must have felt before he, or she, was taken into a theatre such as that at Old St Thomas's for a major operation that was to be carried out without anaesthetics or antiseptics of any kind.

The best description of one of these harrowing operations, carried out on a fully conscious human being, was written a little later than the period with which this book is supposed to deal. John Brown, author of the unforgettable *Rab and His Friends*, was not born until September 1810, but the scenes he recorded had changed in no respect at all for several decades.

Brown was born in Lanarkshire, in Scotland, like several other successful medical men who have been mentioned in these pages. He was apprenticed at Edinburgh to the celebrated Doctor James

Syme, who was Professor of Surgery at the Scottish capital and, probably, was the cleverest operator of his time in the whole of the United Kingdom. While he was clinical clerk at the Minto House Hospital, Brown observed carefully certain incidents in which a dog named 'Rab' was involved. Brown's writings are, historically, very important, because their poignancy is believed to have made his son-in-law, Joseph Lister, particularly aware of the tragic consequences of septic infection:

... Six years have passed,—a long time for a boy and a dog: Bob Ainslie is off to the wars; I am a medical student, and Clerk at Minto House Hospital ...

One fine October afternoon, I was leaving the hospital, when I saw the large gate open, and in walked Rab, with that great and easy saunter of his. He looked as if taking general possession of the place; like the Duke of Wellington entering a subdued city, satiated with victory and peace. After him came Jess, now white with age, with her cart; and in it a woman, carefully wrapped up,—the carrier leading the horse anxiously, and looking back. When he saw me, James (for his name was James Noble) made a curt and grotesque 'boo', and said, 'Maister John, this is the mistress; she's got a trouble in her breest—some kind o' an income we're thinkin'.'

By this time I saw the woman's face; she was sitting on a sack filled with straw, her husband's plaid round her, and his big-coat, with its large white metal buttons, over her feet. I never saw a more unforgettable face—pale, serious, lonely, delicate, sweet, without being what we call fine. She looked sixty, and had on a mutch, white as snow, with its black ribbon; her silvery smooth hair setting off her dark-grey eyes—eyes such as one sees only twice or thrice in a lifetime, full of suffering, but also full of the overcoming of it; her eyebrows black and delicate, and her mouth firm, patient, and contented, which few mouths ever are.

As I have said I never saw a more beautiful countenance, or one more subdued to settled quiet. 'Ailie', said James, 'this is Maister John, the young doctor; Rab's freend, ye ken. We often speak aboot you, doctor.' She smiled, and made a movement, but said nothing; and prepared to come down, putting her plaid aside and rising. Had Solomon, in all his glory, been handing down the Queen of Sheba at his palace gate, he could not have done it more daintily, more tenderly, more like a gentleman, than did James the Howgate carrier, when he lifted down Ailie, his wife. The contrast of his small, swarthy, weatherbeaten, keen, worldly face to hers—pale, subdued, and beautiful—was something wonderful. Rab looked on concerned and puzzled; but ready for anything that might turn up,—were it to strangle the nurse, the porter, or even me. Ailie and he seemed great friends.

'As I was saying, she's got a kind o' trouble in her breest, doctor; wull ye tak' a look at it?' We walked into the consulting-room, all four; Rab grim and comic, willing to be happy and confidential if cause could be shown, willing also to be quite the reverse, on the same terms. Ailie sat down, undid her open gown and her lawn handkerchief round her neck, and, without a word, showed me her right breast. I looked at and examined it carefully,—she and James watching me, and Rab eyeing all three. What could I say? there it was, that had once been so soft, so shapely, so white, so gracious and bountiful, 'so full of all blessed conditions',—hard as a stone, a centre of horrid pain, making that pale face, with its grey, lucid, reasonable eyes, and its sweet resolved mouth, express the full measure of suffering overcome. Why was that gentle, modest, sweet woman, clean and lovable, condemned by God to bear such a burden?

I got her away to bed. 'May Rab and me bide?' said James. '*You* may; and Rab if he will behave himself.' 'I'se warrant he's do that, doctor'; and in slunk the faithful beast. I wish you could have seen him. There are no such dogs now: he belonged to a lost tribe. As I have said, he was brindled, and grey like Aberdeen granite; his hair short, hard, and close, like a lion's; his body thick set, like a little bull—a sort of compressed Hercules of a dog . . . Rab had the dignity and simplicity of great size; and having fought his way all along the road to absolute supremacy, he was as mighty in his own line as Julius Caesar or the Duke of Wellington; and he had the gravity of all great fighters.

Next day, my master, the surgeon, examined Ailie. There was

no doubt it must kill her, and soon. It could be removed—it might never return—it would give her speedy relief—and she should have it done. She curtsied, looked at James, and said, 'When?' 'Tomorrow,' said the kind surgeon, a man of few words. She and James and Rab and I retired. I noticed that he and she spoke little, but seemed to anticipate everything in each other. The following day, at noon, the students came in, hurrying up the great stair. At the first landing place, on a small well-known black board, was a bit of paper fastened by wafers, and many remains of old wafers beside it. On the paper were the words, 'An operation today. J B *Clerk*.'

Up ran the youths, eager to secure good places: in they crowded, full of interest and talk. 'What's the case?' 'Which side is it?'

Don't think them heartless; they are neither better nor worse than you or I: they get over their professional horrors, and into their proper work; and in them pity—as an *emotion*, ending in itself or at best in tears and a long-drawn breath, lessens, while pity as a *motive* is quickened, and gains power and purpose. It is well for poor human nature that it is so.

The operating theatre is crowded; much talk and fun, and all the cordiality and stir of youth. The surgeon with his staff of assistants is there. In comes Ailie: one look at her quiets and abates the eager students. That beautiful old woman is too much for them; they sit down, and are dumb, and gaze at her. These rough boys feel the power of her presence. She walks in quickly, but without haste; dressed in her mutch, her neckerchief, her white dimity shortgown, her black bombazeen petticoat, showing her white worsted stockings and her carpet-shoes. Behind her was James, with Rab. James sat down in the distance, and took that huge and noble head between his knees. Rab looked perplexed and dangerous; for ever cocking his ear and dropping it as fast.

Ailie stepped up on a seat, and laid herself on the table, as her friend the surgeon told her; arranged herself, gave a rapid look at James, shut her eyes, rested herself on me, and took my hand. The operation was at once begun; it was necessarily slow; and chloroform—one of God's best gifts to his suffering children—was then unknown. The surgeon did his work. The pale face showed its pain, but was still and silent. Rab's soul was working within him; he saw that something strange was going on,—blood flowing from his mistress, and she suffering; his ragged ear was up, and importunate; he growled and gave now and then a sharp impatient yelp; he would have liked to have done something to that man. But James had him firm, and gave him a glower from time to time and an intimation of a possible kick;—all the better for James, it kept his eye and his mind off Ailie.

It is over: she is dressed, steps gently and decently down from the table, looks for James, then, turning to the surgeon and the students, she curtsies,—and in a low, clear voice, begs their pardon if she has behaved ill. The students—all of us— wept like children; the surgeon wrapped her up carefully,— and, resting on James and me, Ailie went to her room, Rab following. We put her to bed. James took off his heavy shoes, crammed with tackets, heel-capt and toe-capt, and put them carefully under the table, saying, 'Maister John, I'm for nane o' yer stynge nurse bodies for Ailie. I'll be her nurse, and on my stockin' soles I'll gang about as canny as pussy.' And so he did; and handy and clever, and swift and tender as any woman, was that horny-handed, snell, peremptory little man. Every-thing she got he gave her: he seldom slept: and often I saw his small, shrewd eyes out of the darkness, fixed on her. As before, they spoke little.

For some days Ailie did well. The wound healed 'by the first intention'; as James said, 'Oor Ailie's skin's ower clean to beil.' The students came in quiet and anxious, and surrounded her bed. She said she liked to see their young, honest faces. The surgeon dressed her, and spoke to her in his own short kind way, pitying her through his eyes. Rab and James outside the circle,—Rab being now reconciled, and even cordial, and having made up his mind that as yet nobody required worrying, but, as you may suppose, *semper paratus*.

So far well: but, four days after the operation, my patient had a sudden and long shivering, a 'groofin' ', as she called it. I saw her soon after; her eyes were too bright, her cheek coloured; she was restless, and ashamed of being so; the balance was lost; mischief had begun. On looking at the wound, a blush of red told the secret: her pulse was rapid, her breathing anxious and quick, she wasn't herself, as she said, and was vexed at her restlessness. We tried what we could. James did everything, was everywhere; never in the way, never out of it; Rab subsided under the table into a dark place, and was motionless, all but his eye, which followed every one. Ailie got worse; began to wander in her mind, gently; was more demonstrative in her ways to James, rapid in her questions, and sharp at times. He was vexed, and said, 'She was never that way afore; no, never.' For a time she knew her head was wrong, and was always asking our pardon—the dear, gentle old woman: then delirium set in strong, without pause. Her brain gave way, and that terrible spectacle:

> The intellectual power, through words and things,
> Went sounding on its dim and perilous way;

she sang bits of old songs and Psalms, stopping suddenly, mingling the Psalms of David, and the diviner words of his Son and Lord, with homely odds and ends and scraps of ballads.

Nothing more touching, or in a sense more strangely beautiful, did I ever witness. Her tremendous, rapid, affectionate, eager Scotch voice,—the swift, aimless, bewildered mind, the baffled utterance, the bright and perilous eye; some wild words, some household cares, something for James, the names of the dead, Rab called rapidly and in a 'fremyt' voice, and he starting up, surprised, and slinking off as if he were to blame somehow, or had been dreaming he heard. Many eager questions and beseechings which James and I could make nothing of, and on which she seemed to set her all and then sink back ununderstood. It was very sad, but better than many things that are not called sad. James hovered about, put out and miserable, but active and exact as ever; read to her, when there was a lull, short bits from the Psalms, prose and metre, chanting the latter in his own rude and serious way, showing great knowledge of the fit words, bearing up like a man, and doating over her as his 'ain Ailie'. 'Ailie, ma woman!' 'Ma ain bonnie wee dawtie!'

The end was drawing on: the golden bowl was breaking;

the silver cord was fast being loosed—that *animula, blandula, vagula, hospes, comesque*, was about to flee. The body and the soul —companions for sixty years—were being sundered and taking leave. She was walking, alone, through the valley of that shadow, into which one day we must all enter,—and yet she was not alone, for we know whose rod and staff were comforting her.

One night she had fallen quiet, and as we hoped, asleep; her eyes were shut. We put down the gas, and sat watching her. Suddenly she sat up in bed, and taking a bed-gown which was lying on it rolled up, she held it eagerly to her breast,—to the right side. We could see her eyes bright with a surprising tenderness and joy, bending over this bundle of clothes. She held it as a woman holds her sucking child; opening out her nightgown impatiently, and holding it close, and brooding over it, and murmuring foolish little words, as over one whom his mother comforteth, and who is sucking, and being satisfied. It was pitiful and strange to see her wasted dying look, keen and yet vague—her immense love. 'Preserve me!' groaned James, giving way. And then she rocked back and forward, as if to make it sleep, hushing it, and wasting on it her infinite fondness. 'Wae's me, doctor: I declare she's thinkin' it's that bairn.' 'What bairn?' 'The only bairn we ever had; our wee Mysie, and she's in the Kingdom, forty years and mair.' It was plainly true: the pain in the breast, telling its urgent story to a bewildered, ruined brain; it was misread and mistaken; it suggested to her the uneasiness of a breast full of milk, and then the child; and so again once more they were together, and she had her ain wee Mysie in her bosom.

This was the close. She sunk rapidly; the delirium left her; but as she whispered, she was clean silly; it was the lightening before the final darkness. After having for some time lain still— her eyes shut, she said, 'James!' He came close to her, and lifting up her calm, clear, beautiful eyes, she gave him a long look, turned to me kindly but shortly, looked for Rab but could not see him, then turned to her husband again, as if she would never leave off looking, shut her eyes, and composed herself. She lay for some time breathing quick, and passed away so gently, that when we thought she was gone, James, in his old-fashioned way, held the mirror to her face. After a long pause, one small spot of dimness was breathed out; it vanished away, and never returned, leaving the blank clear darkness of the mirror without a stain. 'What is our life? It is even a vapour, which appeareth for a little time, and then vanisheth away.'

Rab all this time had been full awake and motionless: he came forward beside us: Ailie's hand, which James had held, was hanging down; it was soaked with his tears; Rab licked it all over carefully, looked at her, and returned to his place under the table.

James and I sat, I don't know how long, but for some time,— saying nothing: he started up abruptly, and with some noise went to the table, and putting his right fore and middle fingers each into a shoe, pulled them out, and put them on, breaking one of the leather latchets, and muttering in anger, 'I never did the like o' that afore!'

I believe he never did; nor after either. 'Rab!' he said roughly, and pointing with his thumb to the bottom of the bed. Rab leapt up, and settled himself; his head and eye to the dead face. 'Maister John, ye'll wait for me,' said the carrier; and disappeared in the darkness, thundering down stairs in his heavy shoes. I ran to a front window: there he was, already round the house, and out at the gate, fleeing like a shadow.

I was afraid about him, and yet not afraid; so I sat down beside Rab, and being wearied, fell asleep. I woke from a sudden noise outside. It was November, and there had been a heavy fall of snow. Rab was in *statu quo*; he heard the noise too, and plainly knew it, but never moved. I looked out; and there, at the gate, in the dim morning—for the sun was not up, was Jess and the cart,—a cloud of steam rising from the old mare. I did not see James; he was already at the door, and came up the stairs, and met me. It was less than three hours since he left, and he must have posted out—who knows how?—to Howgate, full nine miles off; yoked Jess, and driven her astonished into town. He had an armful of blankets, and was streaming with perspiration. He nodded to me, spread out on the floor two pairs of old clean blankets, having at their corners, 'AG, 1794' in large letters in red worsted. These were the initials of Alison

Graeme, and James may have looked in at her from without—unseen but not unthought of—when he was 'wat, wat, and weary', and had walked many a mile over the hills, and seen her sitting, while 'a' the lave were sleepin' '; and by the firelight putting her name on the blankets for her ain James's bed. He motioned Rab down, and taking his wife in his arms, laid her in the blankets, and happed her carefully and firmly up, leaving the face uncovered; and then lifting her, he nodded again sharply to me, and with a resolved but utterly miserable face, strode along the passage, and down stairs, followed by Rab. I also followed, with a light; but he didn't need it. I went out, holding stupidly the light in my hand in the frosty air; we were soon at the gate. I could have helped him, but I saw he was not to be meddled with, and he was strong, and did not need it. He laid her down as tenderly, as safely, as he had lifted her out ten days before—as tenderly as when he had her first in his arms when she was only 'A.G.',—sorted her, leaving that beautiful sealed face open to the heavens; and then taking Jess by the head, he moved away. He did not notice me, neither did Rab, who presided along behind the cart.

I stood till they passed through the long shadow of the College, and turned up Nicolson Street. I heard the solitary cart sound through the streets, and die away and come again; and I returned, thinking of that company going up Liberton brae, then along Roslin muir, the morning light touching the Pentlands and making them like on-looking ghosts; then down the hill through Auchindinny woods, past 'haunted Woodhouselee'; and as daybreak came sweeping up the bleak Lammermuirs, and fell on his own door, the company would stop, and James would take the key, and lift Ailie up again, laying her on her own bed, and having put Jess up, would return with Rab and shut the door.

James buried his wife, with his neighbours mourning, Rab inspecting the solemnity from a distance. It was snow, and that black ragged hole would look strange in the midst of the swelling spotless cushion of white. James looked after everything; then rather suddenly fell ill, and took to bed; was insensible when the doctor came, and soon died. A sort of low fever was prevailing in the village, and his want of sleep, his exhaustion, and his misery, made him apt to take it. The grave was not difficult to re-open. A fresh fall of snow had again made all things white and smooth; Rab once more looked on and slunk home to the stable . . .

8

A Dose of the Pox

. . . Outward be fair, however foul within;
Sin if thou wilt, but then in secret sin . . .

CHARLES CHURCHILL, 1731–64

Venus—the beautiful goddess, in ancient times, of fertility and love—has given her name to a group of the most unpleasant diseases men (and women) can contract. The group includes syphilis, destroyer of body and brain, which William Shakespeare almost certainly had in mind when he included this acrid piece of dialogue in the scene, in *Hamlet, Prince of Denmark*, in which two clowns are digging a grave for poor drowned Ophelia:

> *Hamlet*: How long will a man lie i' the earth ere he rot?
> *First Clown*: Faith, if he be not rotten before he die—as we
>   have many pocky corses now-a-days, that will scarce hold
>   the laying in—

It includes also gonorrhoea, the germs of which multiply at an enormous rate, spreading to all the glands and crevices of the mucous membrane of the urethra and other passages, producing so much inflammation, and pain, that the patient may be unable to move about.

A venereal disease of one kind or another—probably gonor-rhoea—must have been a serious trouble as far back as the days of Moses, who could think of no better treatment for it than putting the sufferer to death. At least one pope—Ubertinus VIII—is said to have died of a venereal disease and, according to a manuscript preserved at Lincoln College, Oxford, John of Gaunt, who died in 1399, met his end through 'putrefaction of the genital member due to the performance of carnal congress with women'. The physical, mental and moral degeneration of many noblemen during the reigns of the Tudor, Stuart and Hanoverian sovereigns can be fairly safely ascribed to the onset of syphilis.

No one can say exactly when it was first established that there was any significant connection between the diseases of Venus and the act of procreation, though we do know that by the twelfth century AD bye-laws were being passed in many parts of Europe which forbade male citizens to have anything to do with whores who were suffering from 'the burning'. The discovery that there might be several entirely different maladies that were propagated 'under the aegis of Aphrodite' was made more recently, even, than that. During the eighteenth century, gonorrhoea, soft chancre and syphilis were all usually lumped communally together under some such label as 'the foul disease', or, more colloquially, 'the pox'.

It is often said that the syphilis germ or spirochete was brought to Europe, or was brought back to Europe in a revitalized and more active form, by Christopher Columbus's sailors, early in 1493, when the great explorer returned to Spain from the newly dis-covered 'Asian' islands. By April of that year, it is known, fierce epidemics of an acute venereal disease were raging in the north and south of Spain. From there, the armies of Charles VIII took the trouble with them when they marched to Florence, Siena, Rome and Naples. By the beginning of the sixteenth century, the 'great pox'—as some called it—was sweeping like an unleashed tornado through all the charted parts of the world. The name by which it became most generally known—*morbus gallicus*, or 'The French disease'—suggests that Spain's great neighbours were not, in those far-off days, any more universally popular than they are today.

For more than four centuries after Columbus returned with his seriously infected sailors from the 'Asian Isles', the cause of the French disease—the tiny, corkscrew-shaped organism known now as *spirocheta pallida*—remained unidentified. Many other possible causes were suggested. William Clowes, surgeon at St Bartholo-mew's Hospital, London, in 1579 published his own provocative views:

> ... It is wonderfull to consider [he wrote] how huge multi-tudes there be of such as be infected with [the disease called

morbus gallicus] and that dayly increase to the great daunger of the common wealth and the stayne of the whole nation: the cause whereof I see none so great as the licentious and beastly disorder of a great number of rogues and vagabondes: the filthye life of many lewd and idell persons, both men and women, about the citye of London and the great number of lewd alehouses, which are the very nests and harbourers of such filthye creatures: by means of which disordered persons some other of better disposition are many tymes infected and many more lyke to be, except there be some speedy remedy provided for the same . . .

Among every twenty diseased persons taken in to St Bartholomew's Hospital at that time, fifteen would have 'the pockes', claimed William Clowes:

. . . Good poor people be infected by unwary eating or drinking or keeping company with those lewd beasts [he continued] and which either for shame will not bewray it or for lack of good chirurgions know not how to remedy it or for lack of ability are not able otherwise to provide for the cure of it . . .

An excess of copulation, even between the same two persons, was regarded by some other doctors as the probable cause of the 'French disease'. In his *Dissertation on the Pox*, published in 1694, the celebrated naturalist Martin Lister advanced the theory that the disease was transmitted to man, in tropical America, by the huge lizard known as the iguana. Lister did not explain whether the iguana fancied the man, or man the iguana.

The possibility that infants might acquire syphilis congenitally —that is, be born with the disease—occurred to medical men as early as the sixteenth century. In 1565 Simon de Vallembert, physician to the Duchess of Savoy and Berny, recorded publicly that he had seen a goldsmith at Tours who had had the Great Pox fourteen or fifteen years before, after which he had not felt ill at all. In spite of the man's apparent return to health, all his children had developed the pox within seven or eight days of their birth, and had given the malady to their nurse:

... Although the mother was an honest woman well spoken of, who strangely enough had never taken the disease from her husband and had not been affected in any way ...

François Mauriceau devoted a whole chapter of his book on midwifery to the question of *How to cure the Venereal Lues in Infants*. Henry Bracken, who published the popular *Midwife's Companion* in 1737, thought that Mauriceau had been talking a load of nonsense. He observed, dryly:

... Monsieur Mauriceau is of Opinion that a Child afflicted from the Nurse, or bringing the French Disease, as 'tis called, into the World with it, is capable of infecting whole Families and says such things have been often seen: but really I think this ingenious Frenchman talks a little too far with regard to his National Disease, for I am well persuaded that although this Distemper is of the contagious or infectious Tribe, yet that it is communicated in such sort, as many Authors fondly imagine, is meer Stuff ... Therefore I am positive (though a great many bad People would screen themselves by saying they are infected by the Child's sucking their Breasts) that the Venereal Lues, French or Neapolitan Disease, call it which you will, is not many Times, nay very rarely communicated otherwise than by Coition ...

It is difficult to tell from the Bills of Mortality that have survived just how many sufferers from venereal diseases actually died, during the seventeenth and eighteenth centuries, as a direct result of their complaints. In some *Observations* published in 1662, John Graunt, the English statistician, questioned the accuracy of the Bills, particularly where the 'French pox' was concerned. In 229,250 deaths, he said, 'we find not above 392 to have died of the pox.' It was not good, he suggested, to let the world be lulled into a security and 'belief of impunity' by the Bills, which were intended not only to be as 'Deathsheads to put Men in mind of their Mortality, but also as Mercurial Statutes to point out the most dangerous waies that lead us into it and misery'. So he proceeded to point out the pox's unacknowledged dangers:

... Forasmuch as by the ordinary discourse of the World it seems a great part of Men have at one time or other had some species of this Disease I, wondering why so few died of it, especially as I could not take that to be so harmless whereof so many complained very fiercely: upon inquiry I found that those who died of it out of the Hospitals, especially that of Kingsland and the Lock in Southwark, were returned to [ie certified as having died from] Ulcers and Sores. And in brief I found that all mentioned to dye of the French Pox were returned by the Clerks of St Giles's and St Martin's in the Fields only, in which place I understood that most of the vilest and most miserable Houses of Uncleanness were: from whence I concluded that only hated persons and such whose very Noses were eaten off were reported by the Searchers to have died of this too frequent Malady ...

The authorities were quite pleased to have the high incidence of venereal diseases played down in this way. It did no country any good, on the international scene, to have its most serious in-built weaknesses too obviously displayed.

The methods by which venereal diseases were treated prior to the year 1700 ranged from the absurd to the madly dangerous.

Of course, sufferers from the pox were bled, purged, blistered, and given a variety of emetics, as they would have been if they had contracted any other disease. In addition, they might have been thrashed soundly—as a punishment for having conducted themselves in an unseemly way, and to discourage them from ever doing the same thing again—or they might have been subjected to some entirely useless old wives' remedy—in a few places, a pox-ridden man would have had his penis wrapped in the warm, steaming parts of a fowl that had just been torn asunder, while it was still alive.

More fortunate patients would have been treated with mercury, or with guiac.

No one knows exactly when the therapeutic qualities of mercury first became known to physicians and surgeons, but there is certain evidence that mercurial salves were recommended for skin eruptions of various kinds right through the Middle Ages. In 1540 Pietro Andrea Mattioli of Siena tried to cure syphilis by administering mercury internally. In the following year Paracelsus, the great medical thinker, met a violent end in a tavern brawl, but in a work published posthumously he expressed his wholehearted approval of Mattioli's methods. For some time after that, mercury was almost universally prescribed, and in some cases had a beneficial effect.

Guiac was made from the bark of a tree that was first introduced into Spain in the year 1508 from the West Indian island of Hispaniola. In its original habitat, the bark of the guiac was used by the natives for treating their own cases of syphilis—it caused violent sweating, they found, and was sometimes effective. By the middle of the seventeenth century the use of guiac had become so fashionable in Europe that mercury, temporarily, went out of favour with the medical profession. (In 1685 the governors of London's St Thomas's Hospital resolved that 'the ancient guiacum diet drink and no other is to be given to patients with the foule disease, or French pox, unless the physicians order other . . . ') Then, as the seventeenth century ended, mercury entirely regained its popularity with the medical profession, and was not to lose its prime importance until long after the eighteenth century was over. The crude students' jest—'A moment with Venus may mean a lifetime with Mercury'—has only quite recently lost its significance.

Patients suffering from venereal diseases who are taken into hospital are bound to present some exceptional problems. In St Bartholomew's and other London hospitals during the eighteenth century, patients known to have 'foul' diseases were carefully segregated from other inmates who—to repeat the surgeon William Clowes's words—'might be infected by unwary eating or drinking or keeping company with those lewd beasts'. The Orders of St Thomas's Hospital, posted up in the wards in 1752, included this intimidating paragraph:

> . . . XXVIII. Item, That Patients admitted into this House, who have the Foul Disease, shall knowingly or wilfully conceal the same at the time of Taking-in, and shall be placed in a Clean Ward, every such Patient when discovered shall be immediately discharged the House . . .

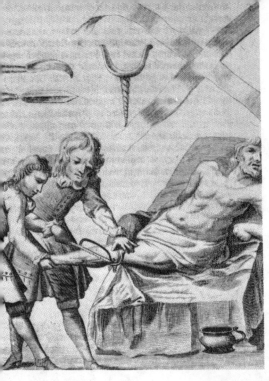

The Amputation, from the German book *Chirugea Curiosa* by M. G. Purmann, 1716.

Doctors setting a limb, from an engraving by Penzel, 1784.

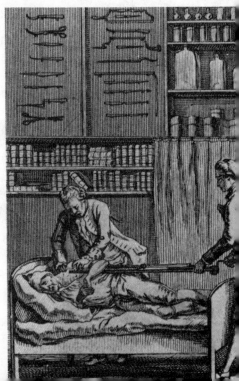

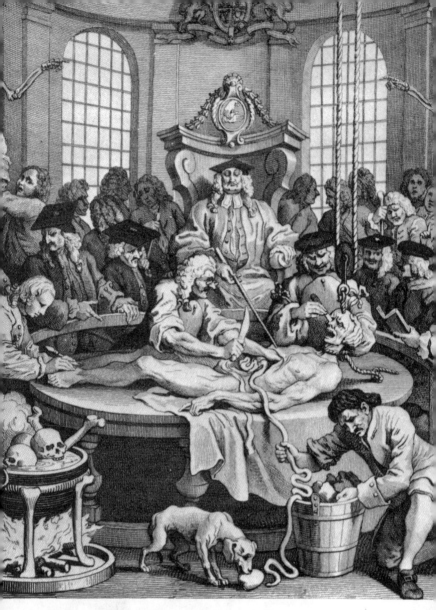

Hogarth's *The Reward of Cruelty*, 1751. Otherwise known as *The Post Mortem*, this is Hogarth's caricature of the medical profession.

'Foul' patients had to pay more for the treatment they received, and for their accommodation, than 'clean' patients. And why not? They were there, as a direct result of their own self-indulgence, and were being divinely punished, most people believed, for their immoral conduct.

Unfortunately for the hospital authorities, the extra cash this decision brought in to their coffers was a serious embarrassment. It might be unwise, the governors of St Thomas's thought, to advertise the fact that the hospital was taking money, tainted money, for interfering with a decree of Providence. If they made too much of this unexpected stroke of good fortune, potential benefactors of a devout frame of mind might be discouraged from remembering the hospital in their wills. So the governors— being, in the main, wise City men—ordered in July 1789 that in future no returns should be made of the admission fees paid by 'foul' patients. It would be better for everyone concerned, they decided, if the money taken from the venereals dropped silently and discreetly into the till.

During the whole of the eighteenth century, patients in the 'foul wards' of hospitals were liable to be subjected to the almost unbearable ordeal known as 'salivating'.

This prolonged operation—carried out, of course, without any form of anaesthetic—came into favour with the medical profession during the later decades of the previous century, just before the use of the guiac bark lost its appeal. (On 7 June 1670, it is recorded in the minutes, the governors of the old St Thomas's Hospital ordered that 'stoves should be prepared for the sweating of venereal patients'.) In that hospital two wards—the Lazarus and Susannah wards—were used for salivating. The old Lazarus ward was partly underground, however, and very damp. In the year 1704 it ceased to be used for salivating and was turned into an engine house. Another ward was found for the purpose, with hot baths already in position.

Richard Austin's case book, written at St Thomas's Hospital in 1725 when Austin was a pupil there, contains a detailed description of 'a salivation'. First comes Austin's summary of the basic principles of the process:

. . . A salivation is caus'd by some of ye preparat. of Mercury and tis the saline particles of calomel that vellicates [makes to twitch, or move convulsively] ye fibres of ye Stomack so as to discharge its contents, and thereby part of ye salts fixes upon ye glands of ye mouth and causes a salivat . . .

A salivation could be raised either by the internal application of mercury or by the external application of a mercury ointment, noted Austin. Either way, it would be 'begun & ended by ye Apoth. Mr. Dickman, according to ye humour of ye Doctor & Surgeon'. The most common way, he said, was by the use of an ointment, 'particularly when ther's any Eruption, pains & diseas'd bones.'

The unfortunate patient to whom this grim form of treatment was recommended would be fitted out, first, with a suit of thick flannel. Then, he would be provided with a quantity of mercury ointment, and with it he would be required to 'annoint every part for three nights except Breast, Belly and Back for fear of a paralysis by offending ye nerves'. On the fourth day the patient would be required to rest so that the effects of these applications could be studied.

Mr Paul, one of the three surgeons attached to St Thomas's Hospital at that time, thought that the 'commonness of the thing makes 'em do it so promiscuously and with such indifferency that it is a very uncertain way'. Mr Paul ordered his patients to apply the mercury ointment more exactly. On the first night—he directed his charges—they should anoint, with the prescribed quantity of ointment, their legs and feet only. On the second night, they should anoint their thighs; and on the third, their arms. On the fourth day they should rest, according to the accepted practice, but after that they would be required to take the mercury internally.

. . . This is done [recorded Richard Austin] before ye fire & ye patients immediately put on woolen stockings flannen [flannel] shirt & drawers & flannen round ye Neck, and from ye first night keep there bed all ye while, the patient is carefully supplied with Hfs [draughts] of warm broth, gruel or Bear [beer] every hour or two.

Some begin to spit and ye gums swell after ye first or 2nd

night, & by raising it gently at first, tis easy to know whether more be requir'd, he must first abstain from flesh & eat nothing but what's simple & easy to digest.

Each patient is furnished with a bellyed pot which holds a pint not unlike a syrup pot, all close at Top excepting a little round hole for ye saliva to run. They seldom sleep above 2 or 3 hours at a time, nor ought they to lay on their Backs least [lest] they swallow ye saliva, or hang their face over ye Pots, as they often do that has a continuall dribling, for t'will make ye face swell. Chancres are usually cut off with sissars or where they grow in Clusters are par'd off before they lye doen & then are allways annointed well which commonly cures 'em.

Nodes are frequently resolv'd by it & assisted by Emp. Mercuriale [mercury ointment], but if they be very painfull are laid open by Caust. [cautery] during salivat.

Buboes are either Suppurated, or destroyed by Caust & towards ye end of ye work a Salivat. compleats ye cure.

Carious bones will sooner exfoliate dureing a salivat. than otherwise . . .

Mr Ferne—another of the surgeons working at St Thomas's Hospital while Richard Austin was there as a pupil—seems to have preferred the internal administration of mercury to external anoinment. He used to prescribe a daily bolus, or pill, which contained fifteen grains of calomel, varying this occasionally with a 'red bolus' (ten grains of anti-syphilitic powder, or mercury sulphide). This drastic treatment was to be continued for twenty-five days, the wretched patient spitting out $2\frac{1}{2}$ to 3 pints of saliva each day and finding, eventually, that all his teeth were loose. At the end of this treatment—it may on occasions even have been a cure—he was allowed to 'spit off all' and given a final purge.

In spite of all the salivation that was carried out during the eighteenth century, and in spite of all the teeth that were spat out into bedside pots, venereal diseases continued to rampage. The Russians were particularly hard hit by them, owing, it was said, to the disgustingly dirty conditions under which all classes there lived. Peter the Great of Russia, King Christian VII of Denmark, King Frederick II of Prussia and many other notable and responsible people are believed to have been fundamentally affected, in their behaviour as well as in their health, by the ubiquitous spirochete. In 1785 the Portuguese specialist Antonio Sanchez published an urgent warning about syphilis:

... It is more widespread than ever [he wrote], and shows its prevalence in the infinite multitude of chronic maladies from which we suffer today, the shrinking of the race in stature and the decay of individual robustness, so frequently to be observed in large cities and seaports. It is amazing and pitiable to see, at every step one takes, so many who are disfigured by ocular lesions, scrofula, malformations of the shoulders and the spine, with crooked legs, meagre frames, wasted flesh and fragile bones. In the face of this evidence I am told that venereal disease is diminishing and that we may soon see it vanish like leprosy. I answer that this malady will only end with the human race itself and that it will be one day the cause of such a revolution in Europe as once overthrew, in the fifth century, the dominion of Rome, that crumbled into dust as the result of physical weakness, luxurious living and the depravity of morals ...

Sanchez had good reason to be alarmed. In the year in which he wrote the words quoted above, the vast majority of the European settlers in Canada were found to be suffering from syphilis. In Scotland, where the disease had been taken by Oliver Cromwell's Puritan soldiers, the growths known as 'sibbens', or strawberries, were spoiling the complexions of great numbers of the natives, even, due to heredity, of some clean living natives. Before the end of the century, there were shocking epidemics in Austria, Denmark, the German states, and Norway. The Bishop of Aarhus, in 1792, was appalled by the appearance of the members of his flock who managed to reach the steps of his altar. Many of them, he said, were 'noseless'.

The history of the prevention and treatment—or non-prevention and non-treatment—of venereal diseases during the eighteenth century may have been tragic, but it does contain one short hopeful chapter. What we might call now 'a real breakthrough' came when a citizen of London named Condom invented, somewhere around the year 1750, those invaluable little envelopes known, subsequently, in England as 'French letters' and, on the other side of the Channel, as *'Capotes Anglaises'* or 'English overcoats'.

Mr Condom's prophylactic aids were made—according to the Paris specialist François Swediaur, who advocated their use—from the blind guts of lambs. The intestines were first washed and dried, and then made supple by being rubbed between the palms of the hands with bran and a little almond oil. 'Uniting the advantages of rendering the male organ perfectly secure against infection and that of being seamless', as M Swediaur described them, Mr Condom's ingenious safety devices, prepared and marketed by him with no thought of commercial gain, should have earned the whole-hearted gratitude of all members of the general public, both English and French. Instead, they brought Mr Condom so much discredit and mockery that he was compelled to change his name.

9

Some Eighteenth-Century Spas and Watering Places

. . . Water is best . . .

PINDAR, *c* 522–442 BC

However much the medical men of the eighteenth century might differ in their opinions about diseases, and how diseases should be treated, they were agreed almost unanimously about one thing—practically all of them thought that natural mineral waters had been provided by God, or by some unnamed supernatural being, principally for the purpose of healing mankind, or at least for providing man with some relief from his most distressing discomforts. The places where waters impregnated with minerals oozed, flowed or gushed from the earth's surface were, therefore, regarded with a certain amount of reverence.

This reverence was, in part at least, historic, for spas were called originally 'holy wells'—they were pools and springs to which men and women went when they wished to pray for health. If, afterwards, the patients were cured or relieved, the saints to whom the wells were dedicated were thought, beyond doubt, to have been principally responsible. After the Reformation in England, when the powers of the saints were generally discredited by King Henry VIII's orders, the holy wells became, more tamely, 'wishing wells'. By Oliver Cromwell's time many of the ancient wells had fallen into disuse, but a little of their old prestige lingered on in some dim folk memory. And some newly-found wells were starting to come into favour.

The waters at Epsom and Tunbridge, to the south of London—for instance—were enthusiastically recommended for their patients by many seventeenth-century doctors. (There was a

Doctor Madan who praised the Tunbridge waters, which, he said, 'with their saponary and detersive quality, clean the whole microcosm or body of man from all feculency and impurities. No remedy is more effecual in hypochondriacal and hysterick fits by suppressing the anathymiasis of ill vapours, and hindering damps to exhale to the head and heart.') These places attracted many citizens from the capital, too—both rich and poor—who found that in such pastoral resorts they could escape from the city's oppressive responsibilities and enjoy themselves in freedom and frivolity.

At the beginning of the period with which we are dealing, no natural springs were more widely renowned and respected in Britain and America than those that had suggested a gloriously appropriate name for Bath, the pleasant little township set in a secluded West of England valley. As far back as the days of the Roman occupation of Britain—and possibly even earlier than that —there had been baths on the spot. When the Romans were there, the settlement had been called Aquae Sulis, the waters belonging to a Celtic god.

The entrance to the Roman baths at Bath had been by way of a courtyard which had a colonnaded walk all round it. In this court were the latrines. In the first room, the visitor undressed. From here, he went into the 'Frigidarium', or cold room. Beyond the Frigidarium lay the 'Tepidarium', moderately heated, and then beyond that again the visitor found the 'Calidarium', or hottest room. In the Calidarium there was a bath of very hot water in which the visitor would immerse himself—being, afterwards, massaged and anointed with oils. Then, having had cold water splashed over the whole of his body, the visitor would return to the Tepidarium, and the course of treatment, or enjoyment, would finish with an exhilarating plunge in the unheated and sometimes extremely chilly waters of the Frigidarium. The whole process would be quite familiar to the Romans who, if they were persons of any consequence, would have had similar baths, though probably on a somewhat smaller scale, in their own villas. What distinguished the baths at Aquae Sulis from all others was the wonderful spring that delivered from the ground, without the need for any underfloor stoves or 'calidaria', half a million gallons of water per day at a temperature of 120° Fahrenheit.

At the beginning of the eighteenth century, Bath's wonderful spring was still pouring forth its goodness, and everyone in England who could afford to enjoy its benefits—aristocrats and squires; politicians and great lawyers; admirals and generals—travelled to it with their ladies and, inevitably, a certain number of attendant parasites. In 1704 the first Pump Room was built, to accommodate the swelling rout of fashionable visitors. In 1708 the first Assembly Rooms were built, a band was engaged to play under the trees in the Grove, and long and enjoyable walks were laid out. Bath was starting to become the leisurely and civilized town that is still so much appreciated today.

From the accounts of many observers we know that the baths at Bath in those days were enclosed in the most rudimentary buildings, all the cisterns—the King's Bath, which measured some sixty feet long by forty feet wide, the Queen's Bath, the Cross Bath, the Hot Bath and the Lepers' Bath—being open to the sky, so that the bathers had no protection whatsoever from the weather. John Wood, in his *Essay Towards a Description of Bath*, published in 1749, wrote of the baths in these words:

> ... Simple cisterns to receive the hot waters of Bath, and contain such quantities as are needed for the purpose of bathing, accommodated with little cells to strip and dress in, and steps to descend from them to the bottom of the water, constitute the public baths of the city in their present state. And the Lepers bath being the place of resource for the most miserable objects that seek relief from the healing fountains, that cistern is proportionately mean, obscure and small: its medium size is no more than about 10 feet in length from north to south, by 8 feet in breadth from east to west; and it is filled by the overflowing water of the Hot bath ...

We know, too, that the baths were only emptied and cleaned at very infrequent intervals. Into the water went people both well and ill, mixed together without any regard to their physical state. (Doctor Robert Peirce, an enthusiastic advocate, claimed that immersions in the Bath baths had cured such diverse afflictions as chorea, green sickness, gout, sciatica, ulcers, uterine diseases, septic wounds, and a host of others.) Many of the dippers would have undergone no other form of immersion for some considerable time and would have been in an unspeakably dirty state when they entered the water. Most bathers stayed in for lengthy periods of time and did not necessarily bother to emerge when they wanted to relieve themselves. Into the water, too, went dead dogs, cats, and many other filthy and decaying items of rubbish for which the less scrupulous inhabitants of Bath had no further use. The impressions formed by the gouty Matthew Bramble, one of the principal characters in Tobias Smollett's novel *Humphrey Clinker*, first published in 1771, are revealing:

> ... Two days ago, I went into the King's Bath, by the advice of our friend Ch——, in order to clear the strainers of the skin, for the benefit of a free perspiration; and the first object that saluted my eye was a child, full of scrofulous ulcers, carried in the arms of one of the guides, under the very noses of the bathers. I was so shocked at the sight that I returned immediately with indignation and disgust. Suppose the matter of those ulcers, floating on the water, comes in contact with my skin, when the pores are all open, I would ask you what must be the consequences?—Good Heavens, the very thought makes my blood run cold! ...
>
> ... But I am as much afraid of drinking as of bathing; for, after a long conversation with the doctor, about the construction of the pump and the cistern, it is very far from being clear to me that the patients in the pump-room don't swallow the scourings of the bathers. I can't help suspecting, that there is, or may be, some regurgitation from the bath into the cistern of the pump. In that case, what a delicate beverage is every day quaffed by the drinkers, medicated with the sweat, and dirt, and dandriff, and the abominable discharges of various kinds, from twenty different diseased bodies, parboiling in the kettle below! ...

Undeterred by the shocking state of the waters offered to them, cultured and distinguished people continued to be drawn to Bath as the proverbial iron filings are drawn to a magnet. Oliver Goldsmith, describing the Bath of his day in his *Life of Richard Nash*, published in London in 1762, painted a detailed picture of a typical visitor:

... The lady is brought in a close chair, dressed in her bathing clothes, to the Bath; and being in the water, the woman who attends, presents her with a little floating dish like a basin; into which the lady puts her handkerchief, a snuff-box, and a nosegay. She then traverses the bath; if a novice with a guide; if otherwise by herself; and having amused herself thus while she thinks proper, calls for her chair, and returns to her lodgings ...

According to John Doran's *A Lady of the Last Century*, published in London in 1873, the Cross Bath was primarily reserved, during the eighteenth century, for members of the aristocracy and the 'quality'. Of this bath, he said, the celebrated beauty Mrs Montagu had written:

... Handsome japanned bowls floated before the ladies, laden with confectionery, or with oils, essences, and perfumery for their use. Now and then one of these bowls would float away from its owner, and her swain would float after it, bring it again before her, and, if he were in the humour, would turn on his back and affect to sink to the bottom, out of mere rapture at the opportunity of serving her ...

In view of the septic qualities of the water in which a swain might 'affect to sink to the bottom', it is hardly surprising that Horace Walpole commented unkindly but realistically, in a letter to George Montagu: 'They may say what they will, but it does one ten times more good to leave Bath than to go to it.'

The people who visited Bath during the eighteenth century in optimistic attempts to return to perfect health were expected to conform to a fairly strict, though unhurried, routine. Most of them would start the day's activities between 6 am and 9 am by taking a bath, either in the King's Bath or the Cross Bath. After that, the patients would normally take breakfast, either in their lodgings or in the Assembly Rooms. After breakfast, those who had already bathed could enjoyably spend their time until 10.30 or 11 o'clock in the Assembly Rooms, taking the waters, or they could go to the Pump Room to watch belated risers taking their immersions. This was, socially, the most desirable meeting place, and was memorably described by Tobias Smollett in *Humphrey Clinker*:

> ... The noise of the music playing in the gallery, the heat and flavour of such a crowd, and the hum and buzz of their conversation gave one the headache and vertigo the first day, but afterwards all these things became familiar and even agreeable ...

The entertainments that were enjoyed in Bath during the long, slow, eighteenth-century evenings were considered by some people to be more splendid, in many respects, than those that could be patronized in the capital, though it is unlikely that most of them would be thought particularly exciting today. There were the balls, for instance, at which interminable minuets were danced, in a rigid and stately fashion, by solitary couples—'a succession of stupid animals', according to Tobias Smollett, 'describing the same dull figure for a whole evening on an area not much bigger than a tailor's shop board.' There were theatres —the first was built in 1705—at which, a Lady Bristol complained, there was 'hardly ever company enough to keep the house warm'. (Later in the century, with Mrs Siddons to be seen in the town in Shakespeare's greatest tragedies, there were more sophisticated dramatic offerings to draw the Bath audiences.) Through most of the century, Bath was a celebrated centre of gambling. By the end of the century, when Napoleon Bonaparte's star was high over Europe, Hannah More, the virtuous authoress, was able to write:

> ... Bath, happy Bath, is as gay as if there were no war, nor sin, nor misery in the world! We run about all the morning lamenting the calamities of the times, anticipating our ruin, regretting the general dissipation, and every night we are running into every excess, to a degree unknown in calmer times ...

The increasing popularity of Bath—and the increasing prosperity of its tradespeople—did not pass unnoticed in other places where there were mineral springs that could be exploited. Town after town, during the eighteenth century, started to advertise that there were healing waters within its boundaries, or within easy walking distance. The vast majority of these places had water so slightly impregnated with any mineral contents that it should not, fairly, have been offered to the public at all and by now most of their feeble springs have been forgotten. Three, within reasonably easy travelling distance of Bath—Cheltenham, Leamington and Malvern—had waters with pronounced purgative qualities that can now be ascribed to the presence of chloride of lime, sodium sulphate, and other chemicals in solution. The first two have 'spa' facilities still. Malvern waters are bottled and sent away to be sold.

In 1773 Cheltenham was little more than a quiet farming village, with only one lodging-house for visitors and two inns, each just large enough to accommodate a few paying guests. The place had one under-used asset, though—it had a spring which, a little more than half a century before, had been seen to leave, where it flowed from some thick clay, a pronounced deposit of salts. The aperient effects of the water from this spring had been known to the local inhabitants for a considerable time. (A Doctor Lucas, who attempted to analyse it, reported that 'he had seen old men drink Cheltenham water by the quart without number, or experimenting [*sic*] any ill effect from so strange a practice, which they had accustomed themselves to on certain days and holidays for upwards of thirty years, without having any disorder, but because they thought it wholesome to cleanse their bodies; therefore observed no rule but to drink it till the water passed clean through them.')

Compared to the gay goings-on at Bath, the entertainments offered at this time to Cheltenham's few visitors were staid and unsophisticated. J Ridley's *Cheltenham Guide*, published in 1781, suggests their limitations:

> ... This public breakfasting is at the Long Room every morning at 10 am during the season, each person pays one shilling. The balls begin every Monday at 8 in the evening and Country dancing closes them at 11. Each person who drinks tea or a dish of chocolate pays sixpense—ladies who dance excepted, the gentlemen their partners paying for them ...

Cheltenham became, suddenly, a place of national importance in 1788 when, on the advice of his doctors—and, perhaps under the influence of Lord Fauconberg, one of his gentlemen-in-waiting, who had a house nearby—King George III, who had been exhibiting disturbing symptoms, travelled to the little Gloucestershire spa and spent five weeks in the town. With the king went Queen Charlotte and three of their daughters.

The royal visit immediately stimulated the development of Cheltenham, since it drew a large number of people to the town, and it made the place, for a short time, the centre of fashionable attention. The king's party found the newly built Fauconberg House—lent for the monarch's use during his stay—rather a squash after the more splendid residences to which they had been used. 'How we shall all manage, Heaven knows,' Fanny Burney recorded in her diary (she had travelled, to be in attendance on Queen Charlotte). 'Miss Planta and myself are allowed no maid; the house would not hold one.'

But there were compensations. Fauconberg House was 'situated on a most sweet spot', Miss Burney wrote appreciatively. She described her arrival there in some detail:

... When we have mounted the gradual ascent on which the house stands, the crowd all around it was as one head! We stopped within twenty yards of the door, uncertain how to proceed. All the Royals were at the windows; and to pass this multitude—to wade through it, rather—was a most disagreeable operation. However, we had no choice: we therefore got out, and leaving the wardrobe-women to find their way to the back-door, Miss Planta and I glided on to the front one, where we saw the two gentlemen, and where, as soon as we got up the steps, we encountered the King. He inquired most graciously concerning our journey; and Lady Weymouth came downstairs to summon me to the Queen, who was in excellent spirits and said she would show me her room.

'This, ma'am!' cried I, as I entered it—'Is *this* little room for Your Majesty?' 'Oh stay,' cried she, laughing, 'till you see your own before you call it little!' Soon after, she sent me upstairs for that purpose; and then, to be sure, I began to think less diminutively of that I had just quitted. Mine, with one window, had just space to crowd in a bed, a chest of drawers and three small chairs ...

In her *History of Cheltenham*, published in 1965, Gwen Hart records that the king kept a reasonably strict routine during his stay at the little spa, reaching the well at six o'clock on most mornings to drink his first glass of the purgative water. The queen and the princesses usually accompanied him at this early hour and walked with him under the elms until the party returned to breakfast at half past seven. Much of the day was spent in walking or riding; dinner was between four and five, and at seven o'clock they appeared again in the Walks or paid calls on their friends staying in the town. On three occasions they visited the little theatre. Sometimes they watched their servants playing cricket in the field near Fauconberg House, since King George, afraid that they would not have enough exercise, had sent for cricket bats and balls for them.

Almost entirely unappreciated in 1700, Malvern started to attract visitors to its tiny 'spa' towards the middle of the century. The man principally responsible for launching Malvern as a centre of healing—Doctor John Wall—was born in 1708 and became, when he was qualified, one of the original physicians at Worcester Infirmary. When he was about thirty-five years old, Doctor Wall tried, in company with one of the Worcester apothecaries, to analyse some samples of the Malvern water. In 1757 he published the results of these experiments, appending an account of several miraculous cures which, he said, could be safely ascribed to the quality of the Malvern water. 'The efficacy of this water seems chiefly to arise from its great purity,' he went on, adding that his analyses showed that there was very little mineral matter in the samples he had taken. A comic couplet quickly went the rounds:

The Malvern water, says Dr John Wall,
Is famed for containing just nothing at all

Benjamin Stillingfleet, who visited Malvern in the summer of 1757, found difficulty in getting a lodging, as the place was so very full. 'Nor do I wonder at it, there being some instances of very extraordinary cures in cases looked on as desperate even by Dr Wall,' he wrote. 'The cures at Malvern could be largely ascribed, he did not doubt, to the fresh air and exercise that visitors were compelled to take in their search for health, the wells being more than two miles from the town and accessible only to those on foot. By 1781 the waters, which had somehow acquired a reputation for being good for healing sore or weak eyes, were being advertised and sold in London at one shilling a bottle. When Cheltenham increased enormously in popularity after the king's visit, Malvern served as an overflow.

Although Leamington did not really come into its own until the reign of Queen Victoria, the twin springs at the little town two miles from Warwick were mentioned in Camden's *Britannica* as early as 1586. During the eighteenth century the springs were almost completely neglected by the lord of the manor who owned them and they were, therefore, largely unused except by the occasional visitor who had been bitten by a mad dog and who had heard that the local waters were better than most for this unusual complaint.

On a January day in 1784, though, William Abbotts, proprietor of Leamington's Black Dog Inn, happened to be standing with one of his neighbours when they noticed bubbles rising to the surface of some water that had collected in a ditch on Abbotts' land. With his cupped hands, the publican's friend took up some of the water, and tasted it. The water had a strong flavour of minerals. Abbotts then fetched a cup and, after sipping the water, agreed that it had an unusual taste. Neither of the men was an expert on spa waters, so Abbotts sent a sample for analysis to Doctor Ker, the principal physician in Northampton. Doctor Ker, after examining the water and submitting it to a few rudimentary tests, praised it highly so Abbotts quickly proceeded to build a bath house on the site and a new hotel in the immediate proximity. By 1794 a Doctor Lambe had declared—in the *Memoirs of the Manchester Philosophical Society*—that the new watering-place, though small, was 'likely to cast Bath and every other Spa into the shade'. Lambe's forecasts were published so widely that three duchesses arrived, separately, to take the newly fashionable waters in a single season. Within ten years, the little hamlet had grown so rapidly that a foreign visitor—Count Puckler-Muskau, from the Court of Bavaria, was able to describe Leamington as 'a rich and elegant town, containing ten or twelve palace-like inns, four large bath-houses with Colonnades and gardens, several libraries, with which are connected card, billiard, concert and ballrooms (one for six hundred persons), and a host of private houses, which are almost entirely occupied by visitors and spring out of the earth like mushrooms'. By 1840—thanks, almost entirely, to the enterprise of William Abbotts—the permanent population of Leamington had risen to upwards of twelve thousand souls. In the spa-visiting season, of course, the town's population was a lot higher than that.

The few significant spas that operated in the north of England in the eighteenth century were used principally, if not entirely, for medicinal purposes, rather than for indulgence—the austerities and discomforts of the towns in or near which the waters surfaced saw to that.

Buxton, set high up in the cold, bare, wind-swept hills of Derbyshire had, and has, thermal waters that were once enjoyed by the Romans, like those of Bath. The place was famous, even in the reign of Queen Elizabeth I. 'Buxton is a *shocking* place, but the blessing of health is worth a state of trial,' wrote Mrs Delany in 1776 to the Duchess of Portland. The spa—far from any other sizeable town—could be reached only by a long and difficult journey, and apartments, when the spa was reached, were hard to find, barely furnished, and, as often as not, infested with bugs. It was the second Duke of Devonshire, comparatively late in the century, who decided to rebuild Buxton in a style so classical and dignified that it would eventually rival Bath in popularity and convenience.

The acid or 'tart' fountain at Harrogate in Yorkshire had been discovered, and the little town had been dubbed 'The English Spa'—after the better-known Belgian watering-place—before the sixteenth century ended. During the seventeenth century the reputation of this medicinal spring set 'upon a rude barren moore' grew steadily. By 1650 a sulphur spring had also come into use in the town. Among the distinguished visitors who travelled to the place was John Ray, the naturalist, who wrote in his diary in 1661: 'We went to the Spaw at Harrogate and drunk the water. It is not unpleasant to the taste, somewhat acid and vitriolick. Then we visited the sulphur well, whose water, though it be pellucid enough, yet stinks noisomely, like rotten eggs.'

Matthew Bramble, in Tobias Smollett's *Humphrey Clinker*,

described the hot baths at Harrogate, as they were in the middle of the eighteenth century, in these uninviting terms:

> ... I was conducted into a dark hole on the ground floor, where the tub smoaked and stunk like the pot of Acheron, in one corner, and in another stood a dirty bed provided with thick blankets, in which I was to sweat after coming out of the bath. My heart seemed to die within me when I entered this dismal bagnio, and found my brain assaulted by such insufferable effluvia ... After having endured all but real suffocation for above a quarter of an hour in the tub, I was moved to the bed and wrapped in blankets. There I lay a full hour panting with intolerable heat ...

The tubs to which Smollett referred were long narrow vessels that were (appropriately) not unlike coffins in shape. In *A Season in Harrogate*, published in 1811, a visitor is made to say of one of them:

> ... Astonished I saw when I came to my doffing,
> A tub of hot water made just like a coffin,
> In which the good woman who attended the bath,
> Declar'd I must lie down as straight as a lath,
> Just keeping my face above water, that so
> I might better inhale the fine fumes from below.
> 'But mistress', quoth I, in a trembling condition,
> 'I hope you'll allow me one small requisition.
> Since scrophula, leporasy, herpes and scurvy,
> Have all in this coffin been roll'd topsy turvy;
> In a physical sense I presume it is meet,
> Each guest should be wrapped in a clean winding sheet?'
> 'Oh, no! my good sir; for whatever's your care,
> You never can catch anything bad in this air;
> And that being settled on solid foundation,
> We Harrogate bath-women spurn innovation.'
> So cavalier like I submitted to power,
> And was coddled in troth for the third of an hour ...

Neither Mrs Hofland, who wrote those lines to amuse, nor Tobias

Smollett, who was also primarily concerned to entertain, were exaggerating. Doctor William Alexander, who published the entirely serious *Plain and Easy Directions for the Use of Harrogate Waters*, said of the sweating bed into which the patient was put, with two blankets below and as many as four blankets above his already perspiring body, as soon as he came out of the bath: 'I would advise all those who intend to go through this process, only to sit down five minutes, and consider, that they are going not only into the same bed, but into the very blankets, where hundreds have lain before them, and where hundreds have not only lain, but sweated; that these blankets must be filled with that sweat; and that it did not arise always from sound and healthful bodies, but from bodies diseased both internally and externally: and if, after these reflections, they can calmly lie down in it, they must have little delicacy.'

Spas and watering places in countries on the continent of Europe during the eighteenth century were, on the whole, rather better ordered than those in the British Isles. Besides Spa itself, which was the most fashionable resort on the Continent until 1807, when most of the town was burned down, there were Ems and Schlangenbad in Germany ('Resorted to very much by hysterical patients,' reported Doctor John Macpherson, the great expert on European spas); Carlsbad, set in the precipitous pine-forested hills of Bohemia; and many more. Edwin Lee, writing on *The Baths of Germany* in 1843, commented on the suitability of these and similar places for 'persons whose general health is disordered, without any marked local disease, as is frequently seen in those whose minds are subject to the anxieties attendant on commercial or professional pursuits, and also in those who have been during several months engaged in the routine of metropolitan dissipation'. Having so much to offer the dissipated, who would probably be wealthy as well as discerning, the people responsible for running Europe's spas had little time or use for horrors of the kind to which visitors to Harrogate were compelled to submit.

10

The Insane

. . . Here we come gathering nuts in May . . .

CHILDREN'S SONG

Sir Thomas More, who opposed King Henry VIII on a matter of principle, and who was condemned to death and executed for what some would regard as his strength of mind, and others would call his obstinacy, has been made, in this century, a Saint of the Holy Roman Church.

When he was a younger man, More lived at Crosby Place, near Bishopsgate, on the east side of London—only a few paces from where Liverpool Street Station stands today. Crosby Place, in its grand entirety, has vanished, but the great hall of More's house with its magnificent hammer-beam ceiling has been moved bodily to Cheyne Walk, Chelsea, where it still exists, and is still used daily as a dining-hall in term, by women of the British Federation of University Students.

In his *Four Last Things*, printed in the year 1522 or thereabouts, More said of those of unsound mind:

> . . . Think not that everything is pleasant that men for madness laugh at. For thou shalt in Bedlam see one laughing at the knocking of his head against a post, and yet there is little pleasure therein . . . But what will ye say if ye see the sage fool laugh, when he hath done his neighbour wrong, for which he shall weep for ever hereafter? . . .

More uttered those words, originally, when he was preaching a sermon on the madness of sin. When he mentioned 'Bedlam', he was referring to the Bethlehem Hospital, London's only refuge at that time for the insane, which was only a stone's throw from More's home at Crosby Place. Certainly, More would have seen many mad men, and women, knocking their heads against posts and laughing at the unpleasant consequences. He would have seen the whip used many times, too, in and near the Bethlehem Hospital. The patients in the hospital were not only scourged regularly so that their keepers should be properly respected and protected from violence. The mad inmates were also beaten because physical pain, at that time, was considered to be a thoroughly effective medicine for the mentally disturbed. The dose was to be repeated as often as was necessary.

In his *Apology*, published in 1533, More mentioned a man who had been 'put into Bedlam, and afterwards by beating and correction gathered his remembrances to come again to himself. But, being thereupon set at liberty and walking about abroad, his old fancies began again to fall in his head.' The man behaved in a disgusting way in a number of churches. When More received complaints about this, he made up his mind to cure the lunatic. 'I caused him to be bound to a tree in the street before the whole town, and constables striped him with rods until they waxed weary . . . ' The treatment seems to have met with some success, for More commented: 'Verily, God be thankd, I hear no harm from him now.'

More's profound belief in the value of corporal correction in the treatment of the insane was shared by all but a few enlightened people during the whole of the eighteenth century. The physical punishment might take a number of different forms. At St Nun's Pool, in Cornwall, for instance, the deranged person would be made to stand with his or her back to the water, and then would be thrown suddenly into it. This ducking process would be repeated time and time again, until the patient was half or three-quarters drowned, and thoroughly exhausted. Then, the poor sufferer would be taken to the nearby church, and special masses would be sung. If the ducking-churching sequence did not produce a marked improvement in the mental condition of the person principally involved, he, or she, would be taken back to the water and the 'cure' would begin all over again. The healers at St Nun's Pool were tough, and would not ordinarily give up while any life remained in a patient.

Right up to the year 1793, mad people were immersed in the frigid waters of St Fillan's Pool—a Scottish spring celebrated for its supposed healing powers. Of this pool, Sir Walter Scott wrote, in his long narrative poem *Marmion*:

> Then to St Fillan's blessed well
> Whose spring can frenzied dreams dispel,
> And the craz'd brain restore . . .

After a forced bath in St Fillan's Water, an insane person would be bound hand and foot and left for a night in a nearby chapel. If the patient managed to struggle loose from this desperate bondage during the night, and were still alive next morning, there was some hope—it would be felt—of a cure being successfully effected. Daniel Hack Tuke, sometime President of the Royal Medico-Psychological Association, member of a family famous in the history of lunacy reform, and author of the enlightened *Chapters in the History of the Insane in the British Isles* was not over-optimistic. 'It sometimes happens,' he reported, 'that death relieves him [the patient] during his confinement of the troubles of life.'

The duckers of St Nun's and St Fillan's Pools were, of course, rough and ready though well-intentioned amateurs. From the scholarly Robert Burton's *Anatomy of Melancholy*, first published at Oxford in 1621, modern readers can tell more or less exactly what most professional medical men of Burton's time thought about the causes of insanity and the treatment of the insane. The beliefs Burton quoted were widely held in the following century. As late as 1777, Archbishop Herring was publicly praising Burton's monumental work.

The original cause of madness, wrote Burton, was the Fall of Man. Moral weakness and mental weakness were one and the same thing:

> . . . We are . . . bad by nature, bad by kind, but far worse by art, every man the greatest enemy unto himself . . .

Sin, then, and the machinations of the devil were, according to Burton, the basic causes of insanity. But there were other factors that might help to send a sane man or woman into a state of distraction. Prime among these were six 'non-natural things'—bad air, bad diet, the retention of bodily excretions, too much or too little exercise, emotional disturbance, and lack of sleep:

... Which causeth dizziness of the brain, frenzie, dotage, and makes the body lean, dry, hard and ugly to behold ...

Burton based his idea of the human body, and its physiology, on the teachings of Hippocrates. The most important of the parts contained in the body, Hippocrates had said, were the four humours. If one or more of these humours were present in excess, mental disturbance would result.

So, Burton suggested, the treatment of mental disturbance was quite straightforward. It was just a matter of removing the excess humours from a patient in a speedy and completely effective way. The use of drastic purges, or vomits—referred to, usually, as 'simples'—was in line with current medical practice, and Burton provided a long list of substances that could be hopefully prescribed: antimony, laurel, white hellebore and 'divine, rare, super-excellent tobacco ... A sovereign remedy to all diseases ... But as it is commonly abused by most men ... Hellish, divelish and damned tobacco.' He also recommended aloes, half-boiled cabbage, herb mercury and senna. Most of the medicines he favoured had already been used for many hundreds of years in the treatment of insanity and would continue to be used by country doctors through the whole of the eighteenth century.

Then, the humours that obstinately refused to be purged or vomited away could be evacuated from the outer surface of the body, said Burton. This could be done by blood-letting—either by a surgeon's knife, or by the use of leeches—or by the uncomfortable expedient of raising blisters by applying plasters or hot irons to the skin. 'Cauteries and hot irons are to be used in the suture of the crown, and the seared or ulcerated place suffered to run a good while.' Burton was also keen on the ancient practice of trephining, in which holes were bored in the patient's skull so that the humours that were affecting the brain would be allowed to escape.

Purged, blistered, bled, made violently sick, or burned with red-hot irons—sometimes, treated to all of these drastic expedients—those unfortunate enough to be mentally sick in the eighteenth century did not really stand a good chance of making any kind of a recovery, let alone a complete return to health. So, steps had to be taken to accommodate the insane in such a way that they would be as little nuisance as possible to the rest of the community. This is how it was done.

If the insane person were wealthy or was a member of a wealthy family, he or she might be sent to one of the small private madhouses that are known to have existed at the time. Very high fees were charged at these establishments, but no public or private records of what went on in them appear to have been kept, and as the whole object of the exercise was to confine embarrassing people in conditions of secrecy we are likely never to know. It is probable, though, that the patients were neglected and intimidated, if not treated with outright cruelty. It is probable, too, that a number of patients were wrongfully detained in these places at the instance of relatives who wished them to be conveniently out of the way.

If the insane person came from the poorer classes, he would have to be kept by the members of his family in the best conditions they could possibly manage, and these would usually be pretty bad. If the sane relatives could not cope with the situation at all, the sufferer would probably be turned out of doors and left to wander, distracted and defenceless, like a lost dog or bitch, until he dropped to the ground, never to rise again. In the last resort, the mad person might have to be incarcerated, to ensure greater public security, in the local workhouse or prison.

The 'single lunatic'—that was a term used frequently at the end of the eighteenth century to describe a mad person who was confined alone—would probably be tied or chained in some dark corner of a house or cottage so that he would be prevented from becoming a menace to other people. As late as the year 1807, a Sir G O Peele was moved to write these words to the Secretary of State for Home Affairs:

> . . . There is hardly a parish in which may not be found some unfortunate creature, chained in the cellar or garret of a workhouse, fastened to the leg of a table, tied to the post in an outhouse, or perhaps shut up in an uninhabited ruin; or sometimes he would be left to ramble half-naked or starved through the streets or highways, teased by the scoff and jest of all that is vulgar, ignorant and unfeeling . . .

And, in March 1845, a writer in the *Westminster Review* described the continuing predicament of lunatics:

> ... The portion of the domestic accommodation usually assigned to these unfortunates is that commonly devoted to the reception of coals ... namely, that triangular space formed between the stairs and the ground-floor. In this confined, dark and damp corner may be found at this very time no small number of our fellow-beings, huddled, crouching and gibbering, with less apparent intelligence and under worse treatment than the lower domestic animals ...

The workhouses that existed in Britain in the eighteenth century were institutions intended for the poor. The rich, who had to pay the rates for their upkeep, naturally thought that these places should be run as cheaply as possible. The Guardians of the workhouse in the parish of St George's, Hanover Square, London, recorded with some pride in 1732 that as the result of 'frugality of management under Honourable Persons' they had succeeded in reducing the cost of maintenance of their inmates to the sum of one and ninepence halfpenny per person per week. (Barely sufficient, in today's terms, to keep anyone alive.) The Poor Law authorities at Maidstone, in the county of Kent, announced in the same year that 'A Workhouse is a Name that carries with it an idea of Correction and Punishment'. It is impossible now to assess the number of mentally disordered persons who were housed during the eighteenth century in these harsh and unwelcoming institutions, but it is safe to say that there must have been many thousands. Insane people who committed criminal acts went to gaols and Bridewells in exactly the same way as any other convicted prisoner.

London's Hospital of St Mary of New Bethlehem, mentioned at the beginning of this chapter, was founded in 1247. By 1598 conditions there had deteriorated sadly. The building was situated between two open sewers, and as one of these was usually choked up with filth and full of stagnant water, the inmates had to inhale the poisonous stench of foul drains through the whole duration of their confinement. In addition, the long gallery of the hospital and the dark cells off it had become so filthy that in that year the governors of the Bridewell Prison were forced to admit that the nearby asylum 'was not fit for anybody to enter'. William Shakespeare, who is believed to have spent much of his time in the Bishopsgate area, decided that the 'noxious philtres' required for his most dismal tragedies should be distilled 'from the herbs of Bethlem's garden'.

Thirty years later, the place had gone still further downhill. Donald Lupton, author of *London and the Country Carbinadoed*, who visited the hospital between the years 1629 and 1632, said of it:

> ... It seems strange that anyone should recover here: the cryings, screechings, roarings, howlings, shaking of chains, swearing, fretting, and chafing are so many, and so hideous ...

The crying, screeching, roaring patients were entirely at the mercy of the dishonest stewards of the place, who received the supplies of food and drink sent in by the Mayor and Sheriffs of the City of London, took the choicest bits for themselves, and sold the rest to their helpless howling prisoners for five or six times the real value of the provisions. In 1631, two of the governors paid a surprise visit to the Bethlehem Hospital and found the patients 'like to starve', for they had had 'nothing to eat for days together but some small scraps'.

On 24 January 1674, the governors of 'Bedlam' passed a resolution that:

> ... The hospital-house was old, weak, ruinous, and so small and strait for keeping the great number applying for admission that it ought to be removed and rebuilt elsewhere on some site grantable by the city ...

Four years later, the same governors granted a lease to one William Bates of 'all that old, ruinous and decayed building, lately called the hospital of Bethalem'. The hospital was reconstituted at the nearby Moorfields, to the designs of Robert Hooke. The new building was finished by July 1676.

And very grand it looked, too, by the time it was properly complete. On either side of the imposing front entrance were two colossal statues, which—according to a later official historian of the hospital—were intended to represent two phases of mental disorder: dementia and acute mania. The chained figure on the right of the door was shown drawing in his breath, as if he were about to bellow forth words of anger and menace. The vacant look of the figure on the left was meant to suggest the general paralysis of all energies which precedes dissolution in the last stages of syphilitic collapse. Oliver Cromwell's porter (according to tradition) acted as the model for the figure in chains. The statues were carved out of Portland stone by Caius Gabriel Cibber, father of Colley Cibber the actor and dramatist. In their day, they were considered 'first in conception, and only second in execution, among all the productions of English sculptors'.

Unfortunately for the patients transferred or admitted to the new hospital, though, the accommodation that had been prepared for them by Hooke was noticeably less comfortable than the quarters thought appropriate for the poor creatures who were granted meagre asylum in medieval monasteries.

To the right and left of the entrance hall, in the new Bethlehem Hospital, on both storeys, were long galleries that provided access to the small dark cells in which most of the patients were kept. A few harmless patients, only, were allowed the 'liberty of the gallery'.

The cells were provided with narrow windows—fitted with bars, but with no glass—high up in the back, or south, wall. During the winter months, confinement in these bare and largely unheated chambers would have been, in itself, an exquisite form of torture, even if the patients had been clad in thick woolly clothes. The inmates were not spared any agony, however—most of them, both male and female, were kept throughout the year in a state of nakedness, or in the lightest of shifts. This was ordered, principally, because the authorities could not afford to provide adequate garments with so many patients prone to tearing their clothes to shreds. Straw was provided as bedding for impoverished patients and those who were likely to be unclean in their habits, since it was cheap and could be easily removed from the cells and burned once it had been badly fouled.

In his historical novel *Jack Sheppard*, published in London in 1879, Harrison Ainsworth included a graphic account of the way in which the wilder patients in the Bethlehem Hospital were kept during the eighteenth century. Although Ainsworth's book was a work of fiction, his description may be taken as reasonably accurate, since it was based on evidence given in 1815 by reliable investigators who had found patients confined in the hospital in virtually identical conditions.

Jack Sheppard, a highwayman who is wanted for murder, risks arrest and execution by hanging in his determination to enter Bedlam to see his mother. Mrs Sheppard has been driven to distraction by Jack's violent criminal career:

> ... Jack absolutely recoiled before the appalling object that met his gaze. Cowering in a corner upon a heap of straw sat his unfortunate mother, the complete wreck of what she had been. Her eyes glistened in the darkness—for light was only admitted through a small grated window—like flames, and as she fixed them on him, their glances seemed to penetrate to his very soul. A piece of old blanket was fastened across her shoulders, and she wore no other clothing except a petticoat. Her arms and feet were uncovered, and of almost skeleton thinness. Her features were meagre and ghastly white, and had the fixed and horrible stamp of insanity. Her head had been shaved, and around it was swathed a piece of rag, in which a few straws were stuck. Her thin fingers were armed with nails as long as the talons of a bird. The cell in which she was confined was about six feet long and four feet wide ...

Not much larger than a conventional grave, in fact. And hardly any warmer.

From the day when London's new Bethlehem Hospital was opened, in 1676, the attendants were forbidden by the governors to treat their helpless victims roughly, or to use abusive language in the ordinary discharge of their duties. One of the hospital's physicians—Edward Tyson—actually recommended that the attendants should use 'all the care and tenderness imaginable'. From some memorable paragraphs in Charles Dickens's novel *Martin Chuzzlewit* we can surmise that in spite of Tyson's strictures, the hospital's nurses continued to be drawn, principally, from the rougher classes:

... 'You want', said Mrs Gamp to poor old Chuffey, 'a pitcher of cold water thrown over you, to bring you round; and if you was under Betsy Prig, who has nussed a many lunacies, and well she knows their ways, you'd have it too. Spanish flies is the only thing to draw the nonsense out of you, and if anybody wanted to do you a kindness, they'd clap a blister of 'em on y'r head, and put a mustard poultige on y'r back' ...

Tyson's new idealism started to come to grief when Doctor Richard Hale, who followed kind Doctor Tyson as physician to the hospital, said that he considered 'company' to be 'very beneficial' to the patients, especially to those who were suffering from some form of mental depression. 'Jollity and merriment and even a band of music would contribute to their recovery,' Doctor Hale insisted. So, members of the public were encouraged to visit the long galleries of the hospital on weekdays, and they came in large numbers. The members of the staff of the hospital, finding it agreeable—and profitable—to support Doctor Hale's views, soon announced that if ever a patient did a mischief to himself, or herself, it was always on a Sunday, when visitors were not admitted.

From before the start of the eighteenth century to the year 1770 at least, the Bethlehem Hospital, in London, was one of Britain's principal places of entertainment. During the reign of Queen Anne, Ned Ward, the humorist 'of low extraction', who kept a notorious punch shop and tavern next door to Gray's Inn, said of its visitors:

... The spectators were bad of all ranks, qualities, colours and sizes. There was a Jack to every Jill: people came in singly and went out in pairs. And all I can say of Bedlam is that it is a hospital for the sick, a promenade of rogues, and a dry walk for loiterers ...

The galleries, when the visitors were in, were as jolly and as noisy as any old-fashioned fair. Nuts, fruit and cheesecakes were peddled up and down, and beer was brought in and sold with the full agreement of the patients' keepers. The keepers, themselves, would act as showmen, demonstrating the antics of their 'star' lunatics, and accompanying the performance with some appropriate patter which was often obscene. When William Hutton, a stocking weaver who became an historian, walked in 1749 from Nottingham to London and back, he spent three days tasting the pleasures of the capital at a cost of ten shillings and eightpence. He saw St Paul's Cathedral, the king's home and many other famous sights for free, but he was not altogether satisfied. 'I wished to see a number of curiosities, but my shallow pocket forbade,' he recorded. 'One penny to see Bedlam was all I could spare.' In the hospital, he met 'a multitude of characters' and heard 'a variety of curious anecdotes' and reckoned he had got very good value for his penny.

Occasionally, the happy fairground atmosphere in the Bethlehem Hospital would disintegrate completely. A writer in *The World*, in 1753, reported: 'I saw a hundred spectators making sport of the miserable inhabitants, provoking them into furies of rage . . . ' When that happened, the prisoners would clank their chains and they would drum on the locked doors of their cells in sympathy with the fellow inmates who were being particularly tormented. Within seconds, a general uproar would have spread to almost every part of the hospital.

Only the patients in the last stages of syphilitic deterioration would remain unaffected by a hysterical demonstration of this kind, for these unfortunates, with their spirochete-damaged brains, lived out their latter days in solitary worlds of their own. When William Hogarth composed the eighth scene of the great series of moral paintings he called *A Rake's Progress*, he chose the Incurable Ward of the Bethlehem Hospital as the most appropriate place for his 'hero', Tom Rakewell, to end his wretched career. Tom, who has reached Bedlam by way of the squalid Fleet Prison, has had his head shaved by the prison barber. His ankles, in his new place of confinement, are being fettered by one of the keepers, who is wearing the blue hospital livery. Like most of the other incurables with whom he is incarcerated, Tom is drifting deathwards in torments that are largely of his own making.

Along the rail of the staircase, in this grim picture, Hogarth has painted, in letters so small that they need a magnifying glass to be seen, the words 'Charming Betty Careless'. Betty, who figures in Henry Fielding's novel *Amelia*, was once the queen of London's prostitutes who with her innocent, childlike beauty, turned men, as Circe did, into grovelling swine. One of her victims—presumably the man who has carved her name with such bitter irony on the staircase rail—sits now on the stairs with shaven head and ungartered stockings in the penultimate stage of the disease he has contracted in her bed.

In the year 1728, a Doctor James Monro, who was a son of the Principal of Edinburgh University, became the resident physician of the Bethlehem Hospital. This post carried with it the prime responsibility of the management of the place. In 1752, he was succeeded by his son, John Monro, and after that the office of 'Chief Physician to Bedlam' passed from Monro father to Monro son, in an unbroken line, until 1891.

The control exercised by the members of the Monro family over the medical treatment of the patients in the Bethlehem Hospital was virtually unchallenged from 1728 until the year 1815, when a Select Committee on Lunacy set up by Parliament began its enquiries. For close on a century, the Monros had been arbitrarily imposing on all their patients 'thought to be the proper objects of such evacuations' the discredited techniques recommended by Robert Burton in his *Anatomy of Melancholy*. As Doctor Thomas Monro, giving evidence before the Select Committee was ready to testify:

> . . . Patients are ordered to be bled about the latter end of May, or the beginning of June, according to the weather, and after they have been bled, they take vomits once a week for a certain number of weeks; after that we purge the patients. That has been the practice invariably for years, long before my time. It was handed down to me by my father, and I do not know any better practice . . .

Up to the time of the setting-up of the Parliamentary Inquiry, the Monros had also favoured the generous and indiscriminating use of 'weakening agents'—medicines, that is, which would lower the vitality of the patients to such an extent that any form of violent behaviour would become unlikely. The members of the committee questioned Doctor Thomas Monro about this:

Is there any season of the year when particular medicine is applied?

Yes.

What season is that?

In the months of May, June, July, August and September we generally administer medicines; we do not in the winter season, because the house is so excessively cold that it is not thought proper.

Does that go to them all, male and female?

Yes, not the incurables . . .

Is the medicine administered to the patients on account of their mental derangement, on the consideration of each separate case; or is any general remedy applied?

It is generally given, certainly . . .

Are there a certain number of days in the week in which you bleed, and a certain number of days on which you physic?

All the patients who require bleeding are generally bled on a particular day, and they are purged on a particular day.

And vomited?

Yes, and vomited . . .

All the Monros who reigned at the Bethlehem Hospital prior to the year 1815 favoured the use of mechanical forms of restraint such as straps, shackles and strait-waistcoats when these were deemed necessary. In this, the Monros were merely following the accepted practice of the time. Even the allegedly 'mad' king, George III, was restrained by the Rev Francis Willis, a rural clergyman who, 'from motives of principle and charity towards his fellow creatures' had interested himself in the insane. For thirty years, Willis had kept a private asylum in Lincolnshire in which he had treated patients from good families who could afford his high fees, and—according to his own claims—he had achieved excellent results. The crunch came shortly after Willis was called in by the members of the Privy Council and asked to treat the sovereign for his disturbing symptoms. The courtier Robert Fulke Greville, in his diary, recorded the king's first confrontation with the formidable Willis:

. . . His Majesty received Dr Willis with composure and began immediately to talk to him and seemed very anxious to state to him that he had been very ill, but that he was now quite well again. He told Dr Willis that he knew where he lived, and asked him how many patients he then had with him under his care. He then thus addressed Dr Willis: 'Sir, your dress and appearance bespeaks you of the Church, do you belong to it?' Dr Willis replied: 'I did formerly, but lately I have attended chiefly to physicks [ie medicine].' 'I am sorry for it,' answered the King with emotion and agitation. 'You have quitted a profession I have always loved, and you have embraced one I most heartily detest. Alter your line of life, ask what preferment you wish, and make me your friend . . . '

But Willis was to be anything but a friend of the mentally disturbed monarch. When the king became excited:

. . . Dr Willis remained firm, and reproved him in nervous and determined language, telling him he must controul himself otherwise he would put him in a strait waistcoat. On this hint Dr Willis went out of the room and returned directly with one in his hand . . . The King eyed it attentively and alarmed at the doctor's firmness of voice and procedure began to submit . . .

After he was gone His Majesty continued to abuse the rest of the physicians and now principally as he said for not having dealt fairly with him and by having concealed from him his real situation. After this, the poor dear King, overcome by his feelings, burst into a flood of tears and wept bitterly . . .

In his treatment of the king, Willis was helped by his son, and by a number of strong-arm attendants. Doctors Ida Macalpine and Richard Hunter who, in 1967, published their *George III and the Mad-Business*, which was an entirely new review of the case, described Willis's methods in this way:

. . . So began the new system of government of the King by intimidation, coercion and restraint. No account of the illness from this point on can disregard the King's treatment, and to what extent the turbulence he displayed was provoked by the repressive and punitive methods by which he was ruled. For every non-compliance—refusing food when he had difficulty

in swallowing, no appetite or a return of colic, resisting going
to bed when he was too agitated and restless to lie down, throwing off his bed-clothes during sweating attacks—he was
clapped into the strait-waistcoat, often with a band across his
chest and his legs tied to the bed . . .

Irritants applied by the Willises to the king's legs to raise blisters
proved so painful that the poor monarch, unable to endure
further the agonies they caused him, tore them off. For this, he was
put into the strait-waistcoat again. When he was released, he was
so reduced that he was unable to put his legs to the ground. 'Why
must a king lay in this damn confined condition?' the patient was
heard to say on a later occasion, after a further spell in the waistcoat, lasting nine hours without a break. 'I hate all physicians but
most the Willises, they treat me like a madman.' On being sick,
after being given an emetic, the king was seen to kneel, and heard
to say: 'That he had left undone those things which he ought to
have done, and done those things which he ought not to have
done, and he prayed that God would be pleased either to restore
him to his senses, or permit that he might die directly.' Had the
king not been a man of exceptional strength of body and mind,
suggest Doctors Macalpine and Hunter, he would never have
survived Doctor Willis. It was, they say, 'a triumph of nature over
medicine'.

The rough and ready practices of men such as the Monros and
the Willises did not go entirely uncriticized by their contemporaries. For nearly a century, protests were made—in the
columns of *The World* and *The Gentleman's Magazine*, as well as
from the pulpit—about the severe treatment that was being
meted out to the patients in the Bethlehem Hospital. By 1751
enough people had become conscious of the evils of the place for
there to be a call for some positive action. So, in that year, a new
hospital for the insane—St Luke's—was founded on the north
side of London's Moorfields, and this place was intended to be
organized, as far as possible, on more humane lines than the
nearby 'Bedlam'. The tenth 'consideration' addressed to the
members of the general public and potential subscribers by
the founders of the new hospital was: 'That the patients shall
not be exposed to public view . . .'

When St Luke's Hospital was first opened for the reception of patients, the physician appointed by the governors—a Doctor Battie—was instructed to limit severely the use of bleeding and purging, and he prescribed no medicines more drastic than some mild anti-spasmodics and gentle laxatives. On the whole, the treatment given in the new hospital seems to have been reasonably enlightened, though Doctor Alexander Robert Sutherland, physician to the hospital in 1815, admitted to the members of the parliamentary Select Committee that he very often employed 'the bath of surprise'.

The treatment of the insane in the other countries of Europe during the eighteenth century was hardly any more advanced than the treatment of lunatics in England. In France—to take just one fairly 'civilized' country as an example—the mentally sick were also fettered, and beaten, and given weakening medicines. At the Hospice de Charenton, at St Maurice in Northern France, the inmates were dressed up by their keepers in ridiculous costumes and made to perform simple plays for the amusement of audiences drawn from nearby towns. The first really significant step forward in the treatment of the insane in France was taken by Doctor Philippe Pinel who, in 1792, took the chains off the wretched creatures huddled in the Salpétrière and Bicêtre hospitals in Paris and called on the world to witness the terrible injustices that were being done to this desperately unhappy section of the human race.

In America, the provision of special hospitals for the mentally disturbed lagged a little behind the provision of asylums in Britain and other parts of Europe. In 1751 a petition was sent from the people of Philadelphia, to the House of Representatives. In this petition, the signatories claimed that with the increase of the population of America, the number of the insane had greatly increased. The Philadelphians alleged, too, that some of the insane, 'going at large', were a source of terror to their neighbours who were 'daily apprehensive of the violence they might commit'. So, the Philadelphians asked the House for help in founding a small provincial hospital in which these and other persons suffering from comparable diseases could be safely and comfortably treated. Their request was granted, and the new hospital was opened at Philadelphia in the following year. The building was not designed exclusively for the insane, however. The provision of a public hospital in America for mental cases only did not happen until 1773, when Virginia established a proper asylum. No other public hospital for the insane was opened in America until 1817, when the Society of Friends provided—at Frankford, Pennsylvania—a retreat for the seriously disturbed.

In the hospital at Philadelphia, the famous Doctor Benjamin Rush obtained most of the clinical material on which he based his classic work *Medical Inquiries and Observations upon the Diseases of the Mind* (which appeared, first, in 1812). By the year 1835, Doctor Rush's *magnum opus* had passed through five editions, had influenced an untold number of physicians and surgeons, and was still being studied and acted upon by members of the medical profession whose thinking had not been brought properly up to date, and whose patients suffered almost intolerably in consequence.

One of the first people to suspect that the famous Doctor Rush had unloaded a lot of nonsense on the medico-psychological world was Doctor Daniel Hack Tuke, mentioned earlier in this chapter, who, in the year 1815, crossed the Atlantic in a westerly direction to see what was being done, in his country's lost colony, for the insane. Doctor Tuke, under the influence of Pinel, was already convinced that the whole environment of a mental hospital ought to be therapeutic, and that kindness, freedom of movement and supervised occupation and recreation were essential for the patients. He took one good long look at the work done by his American contemporary and came up with this damning indictment:

... A few passages from his [Doctor Rush's] work will indicate his opinions on the moral treatment of the insane. In mania he recommended the following modes of coercion when milder means had been employed without success:—First, the strait-waistcoat or a chair called the 'tranquillizer', which is another name for the well-known restraint chair; secondly, privation of the patient's customary food; thirdly, pouring cold water into the coat-sleeves so that it might descend down the trunk and body generally; fourthly, the shower-bath continued for 15 to

20 minutes, which one would wish to believe a misprint for seconds. Dr Rush adds that 'if all these modes of punishment fail of their intended effects, it will be proper to resort to the fear of death.' He gives an edifying example of the success of this *dernier ressort*. A certain Sarah T disturbed the whole hospital by her loud vociferations. Light punishments and threats had failed to put a stop to them. The gentleman in charge of the case, Mr Higgins, at last went to her cell and conducted her, loudly vociferating, to a large bathing-tub, in which he placed her. 'Now,' said he, 'prepare for death. I will give you time enough to say your prayers, after which I intend to drown you by plunging your head under this water.' The patient immediately uttered a prayer, such, we are told, as became a dying person; then Mr Higgins, satisfied with this sign of penitence, extorted from her a promise of amendment. We are assured that from that time no vociferations or maledictions proceeded from the cell of Sarah T . . .

The man who had travelled from England to America to investigate the ex-colonials' treatment of insanity noted, with disapproval, that Doctor Rush appeared to like the way Mr Higgins had dealt with this case. The American doctor had commented:

. . . By the proper application of these mild and terrifying modes of punishment, chains will seldom and the whip never be required to govern mad people. I except only from the use of the latter those cases in which a sudden and unprovoked assault on their physicians or keepers may render a stroke or two of the whip or of the hand a necessary measure of self-defence . . .

According to Doctor Rush, the use of cunning could be almost as effective as the use of the whip:

. . . Cures of patients who suppose themselves to be glass [Doctor Rush had written] may easily be performed by pulling a chair upon which they are about to sit from under them, and afterwards showing them a large collection of pieces of glass as the fragments of their bodies . . .

Doctor H F Tuke returned to Europe convinced that one, at least, of the brightest stars in the American medical firmament had been as crazy, at times, as any of the craziest lunatics committed to his care.

II

Quacks and Quackery

*. . . There's ne'er a villain dwelling in all Denmark
But he's an arrant knave . . .*

WILLIAM SHAKESPEARE, 1564–1616

In 1748 a list of popular 'nostrums', or quack medicines, was published in the *Gentleman's Magazine*. The remarks that prefaced this remarkable catalogue of the medicinal codswallop of the day included this illuminating paragraph:

> . . . The rich and the great (generally speaking) will seek relief from the regular physician, and true-bred apothecary; for whom provision is made in the college dispensatory.—But the majority of mankind (in hopes of saving charges, and on a presumption of surer help) are apt to resort to the men of experience, as they are called, whose remedies they are induced to think, from their advertisements (so often repeated, and at so great expense) have been successful in the cure of the several distempers for which they are calculated . . .

The majority of mankind had been resorting to quacks rather than to 'regular physicians' and 'true-bred apothecaries' for a very long time before this. As the seveteenth century had drawn towards its close, the streets of London had been full of such doubtful practitioners as Mrs Norridge, who had been 'left a great secret' by her father, Doctor Duncan, for an 'Infallible Powder', that would dissolve the Stone, and Mrs Nevill, a widow, who lived 'next door to the *Ship*, near the great North Door of St Paul's Church', and who sold Spirit of Wormwood which, she claimed, 'removeth Stitches in the side and disperseth that melancholy water that hinders digèstion'. Most illustrious of all the untrained, uncertified 'healers' at that time were the kings and queens of England and of France.

Almost without exception, until quite recently, English historians and English medical writers have accepted the traditional belief that the practice of 'touching' for the 'King's Evil' —scrofula, or tuberculosis of the lymph glands of the neck— originated with Edward the Confessor (*c* 1003–1066). Unquestioningly, they have gone on re-publishing this hoary old story, claiming that Edward's power to cure the Evil was transmitted by him, hereditarily, to all his successors on the English throne. The French, on the other hand, hold that the English monarchs borrowed from the ancient usage of the kings of France their assumed power to cure by 'the touch'. Macaulay, in his *History of England*, 1860 edition, was inclined to be scornful of the whole business:

> . . . Theologians of eminent learning, ability and virtue gave the sanction of their authority to this mummery; and what is stranger still, medical men of high note believed, or affected to believe in the balsamic virtues of the royal hand . . . We cannot wonder that, when men of science gravely repeated such nonsense, the vulgar should have believed it. Still less can we wonder that wretches tortured by a disease over which natural remedies had no power should have eagerly drunk in tales of preternatural cures: for nothing is so credulous as misery . . .

Mummery it may have been, but the popularity of the ceremony was carefully fostered in England by the Stuart kings for a very good, if selfish, reason: since 'touching' cast the sovereign in the role of one of the Lord's Anointed—demonstrating that he was king by grace of God, and not by the will of his subjects—it helped to restore the declining prestige of the throne. So, Charles I, Charles II and James II touched merrily away, bestowing a gold coin or pendant 'touch piece' on every scrofulous patient who appeared before them. (Their royal generosity led to many of their subjects appearing before them more than once 'for the sake of the gold'.) And the glamour of their practice had a certain transatlantic appeal. In the archives of the town of Portsmouth, in America's New Hampshire, there is a petition which asks the assembly of that province, in 1687, to grant assistance to one of the inhabitants who wanted to make the long voyage to England, to obtain the royal touch.

When James II fled ignominiously from London in 1688, throwing the Great Seal of England into the muddy waters of the Thames as he went, the stranger who came from abroad to sit on the English throne allowed the royal gift of healing, in his adopted country, to fall into disuse. In his *History of England*, Macaulay recalled this:

> . . . William had too much sense to be duped, and too much honesty to bear a part in what he knew to be an imposture. 'It is a silly superstition,' he exclaimed, when he heard that at the close of Lent, his palace was besieged by a crowd of the sick: 'Give the poor creatures some money and send them away.' On one single occasion he was importuned into laying his hand on a patient. 'God give you better health,' he said, 'and more sense.' The parents of scrofulous children cried out against his cruelty: bigots lifted up their hands and eyes in horror at his impiety: Jacobites sarcastically praised him for not presuming to arrogate to himself a power which belonged only to legitimate sovereigns; and even some Whigs thought that he acted unwisely, in treating with such marked contempt a superstition which had a strong hold on the vulgar mind: but William was not to be moved, and was accordingly set down by many High Churchmen as either an infidel or a puritan! . . .

When William of Orange died, and James II's daughter Anne succeeded to the English throne, the new queen decided to revive the practice of 'touching for the Evil'. By doing this, she thought, she would assert her hereditary, God-given right to the Crown, and she would thoroughly discredit the parliament-bestowed right of her predecessor and of the House of Hanover. So, soon after her accession, the Privy Council decided to issue proclamations saying where the queen would perform the miracle. These announcements were read out in all parish churches, and they were printed in the official *Gazette*. In the pages of this journal, one can find graphic reports of the various touchings:

... Bath, October 6, 1702. A great number of Persons coming to this place to be touched by the Queen's Majesty for the Evil, her Majesty commanded Dr Thomas Gardiner, her chief Surgeon, to examine them all particularly, which was accordingly done by him, of whom but 30 appeared to have the Evil, which he certified by Tickets as is usual, and those 30 were all touched privately that day by reason of Her Majesty not having a proper conveniency for the solemnity ...

The form of service used at Queen Anne's 'healings' is recorded exactly in various Books of Common Prayer published during her reign. (One of these prayer books, which is dated '1708 AD', is preserved in the library of the Royal College of Physicians, in London. This book bears the signature of the painter William Hogarth.)

The service would start with a prayer, after which someone would read part of the Holy Gospel according to St Mark, ending 'They shall lay their hands on the sick, and they shall recover'. Then, the Lord's Prayer would be read, and after that all those present would be required to follow these instructions:

... Then shall the infirm persons one by one be presented until the queen upon their knees, and as everyone is presented, and while the queen is laying her hands upon them, and putting the gold about their necks, the chaplain that officiates, turning himself to her majesty, shall say the following:

God give a blessing to this work: and grant that these sick persons, on whom the queen lays her hands, may recover, through Jesus Christ our Lord ...

Backed up by this impressive ritual, the queen's healing touch was eagerly sought for, and before she had been on the throne for many weeks announcements had to be made in the *Gazette* that would get public access to her person properly organized:

... Whereas great Multitudes of People do daily resort to the Serjeant Surgeon's House, and in a very disorderly manner demand to be view'd for the Evil: it is Her Majesty's Pleasure, That all those who are proper Objects do repair only to the

Office appointed at Whitehall for that purpose, where Attendance will be given at convenient Times: of which Publick Notice will be given, Her Majesty having at present thought fit to put off healing for some time . . .

On 30 March 1712, the *Gazette* announced that two hundred people had been 'touched' in St James's Palace, where the queen usually held her public healings. Among that crowd was a small child called Samuel Johnson, who had been brought by his mother from Lichfield, in Staffordshire, on the recommendation of Sir John Floyer, a well-known physician of that town. *An Account of the Life of Dr. Samuel Johnson from his birth to his eleventh year. Written by himself*—still carefully preserved at Lichfield—contains Johnson's recollection of the occasion, in his own distinctive handwriting:

> . . . I was taken in Lent to London to be touched by Queen Anne. I remember a boy crying when I went to the Palace to be touched. I always retained some memory of this journey, though I was then but thirty months old . . .

James Boswell in his *Life of Johnson* gives a fuller account of the infant Samuel's great day:

> . . . Dr Johnson being asked if he could remember Queen Anne, he had, he said, a confused, but somehow a sort of solemn recollection of a lady in diamonds and a long black hood . . .

Boswell says that Johnson's scrofula 'disfigured a countenance naturally well-formed, and hurt his visual nerves so much that he did not see at all with one of his eyes, though its appearance was little different from that of the other'. The great lexicographer carried with him to the grave this unchanging evidence of Queen Anne's ineffectual handiwork.

When George I took Queen Anne's place on the throne of England, the ceremony of healing 'by the touch' became, in his newly-acquired offshore island, virtually obsolete.

Soon after he arrived in London—according to the historian Edward Lathbury—the head of the House of Hanover was asked to 'heal by the touch' the scrofulous son of an English gentleman. The new king refused to do this, telling the English gentleman that he ought instead to consult the exiled Pretender to the English throne, who, as 'James III', was somewhere in Europe. The Pretender, said King George, would be more likely to possess the hereditary healing power of the Stuarts—if, indeed, they had that power at all. The English gentleman took the hint and took his son to France. There, the boy was 'touched' by the Pretender, after which he appeared to recover completely. The gentleman, understandably, became after that a loyal supporter of the Stuart cause.

One Whig lady, mentioned in a book called *London in the Jacobite Times*, published in 1719, scorned the Stuart pretensions and insisted on obtaining for herself the touch of George I:

> ... She made known to the Secretary of State, that she was in a condition of health which would make no progress to one issue till she had kissed the King's hand. The Secretary informed the Sovereign of this womanish caprice, and the good natured monarch laughingly said she might meet him in the Gallery of St James and have her wish gratified. She hung two minutes with her lips to the Royal Hand, King George looking down on her the while in the greatest good humour ...

'Touching' went on, on the Continent, throughout the eighteenth century. Louis XV of France 'touched' no fewer than 2,000 sick persons at his Coronation in 1722. His successor, at his crowning in 1775, performed the ceremony 'in gorgeous apparel' for 2,400 poor sufferers who had been drawn up in tidy rows in the Abbey Park of St Remi. Right to the end of his dissolute life, Charles Edward Stuart was prepared to 'touch' destitute persons who applied to him for the cure of their scrofula. Charles XI, at his coronation in 1824, was the last king prepared to revive the largely discredited ceremonial. With the passing of the French crown to Louis Philippe, the whole ancient pantomime vanished into limbo.

It would be impossible, now, to make a comprehensive list of

the less exalted quacks and mountebanks who achieved notoriety
—and made good livings—during the eighteenth century, for
they were legion. One can only hope to notice, in a book of this
length, a few of the most extraordinary.

For the most part, these unofficial practitioners tended to work
on their own—with, perhaps, one or two assistants or 'barkers'
and, possibly, a monkey or some other captive animal that would
help to attract public attention. (The celebrated 'Doctor' Katter-
felto, at the height of his fame, used to drive round Britain in a
coach drawn by six black horses. He was accompanied on his
journeys by as many as fourteen black cats.)

Among the few who chose to band together were the members
of a company which, at the close of the seventeenth century set up
in London, 'A New Dispensary to save Patient's money and the
Publick Health' in direct opposition to the Institution in Warwick
Lane that had been established by the College of Physicians. The
members advertised their services in this way:

> . . . This Dispensary is not set on Foot by a Society of Physi-
> cians, but is where instead of large Fees, long Bills and Quacks
> more dangerous practice, all persons, in what circumstances
> whatsoever that are curable by physick, may be undertaken and
> managed, with as much safety and judgment and integrity, as
> if they had the advice of a whole Colledge, but with much less
> expense than the meanest pretender. For which purpose the
> Society have provided a Collection of the Choicest Specificks
> yet known, which we call our SECRET CABINET adapted
> to all diseases. Therefore be it known, we have always ready,
> The 'Green Cathartick Elixir', far exceeding any other for
> gripes and cholick; The 'Hysterical Tincture'; The 'Great
> Balsamick Spirit'; The 'White Cardialgick Powder', which in
> all cases excells Crab's eyes, Pearl, Coral and all the Testaceous
> Powders; The 'Grey Ointment' and 'The.Black Cerecloth' or
> Plaister for the Rickets call'd 'The Jewel', a secret left by a
> Famous Jew, who got a vast estate by it, which since his death
> has been communicated to one of the Society as the most
> valuable thing in the World for all wounds.
>
> Note. The Society have taken care to provide particular
> specificks for all the modish diseases . . .

One member of the famous Chamberlen family also claimed to be able to treat most, if not all, of the 'modish diseases'. Paul Chamberlen, born in 1635, was the second son of Peter Chamberlen who will always be associated with the development and use of the obstetric forceps.

Paul Chamberlen's knowledge of the family secret gave him the chance to win fame and to acquire great wealth as an obstetrician. Like his father and his brother Hugh Chamberlen the Elder, though, Paul had a great scheme for the welfare of mankind, and he preferred to devote the greater part of his time and energy to telling the world about it. His project, 'Whereby the Government may be supply'd at all Times with whatsoever sums of Mony they shall have occasion for without Annual Interest and without alienating any more Branches of the Publick Revenue', did not meet with the approval of Parliament, however, and soon it was generally regarded as a nonsense.

Eventually, Paul was persuaded to give up his abortive lecturing and lobbying and he tried, then, to earn fame and a good living by less controversial means. Before long, he was offering the gullible public his 'Celebrated Anodyne Necklaces' which he recommended 'to the world' for 'children's teeth, women in labour, etc'. The necklaces, made of small artificially-prepared beads that looked not unlike barleycorns, were priced at five shillings. In addition to marketing these relatively expensive charms—for they were nothing more—Chamberlen wrote quasi-learned articles about them in various periodicals. Of these literary efforts intended principally to 'puff' the worthless necklaces, the most amusing is *A Philosophical Essay*, which was published in London in 1717. Although this is stated, in the preface, to be the work of an anonymous admirer of Paul Chamberlen, it came, undoubtedly, from the necklace-king's own pen. (With sublime self-assurance, he dedicated the essay to 'Dr Chamberlen and the Royal Society'.) For years after the author's death, all sorts of quack medicines were sold 'up one pair of Stairs at the sign of the Anodyne Necklace next to the Rose Tavern without [outside] Temple Bar'.

A contemporary of Paul Chamberlen's—William Read—operated with great success from an address which was only a few minutes' walk from the Rose Tavern.

Read was born in Aberdeen, and he began his career there as a jobbing tailor. Deciding, quickly, to desert his original calling, Read then took up the far more lucrative trade of quackery. After travelling with his medicinal wares through most of the counties of Britain, he settled in London—at York Buildings, in the Strand—and soon, by persistent advertising, he managed to attract the attention of various influential persons. (In one announcement he made in *The Times*, he said that he had been thirty-five years in the practice of 'couching cataracts, taking off all sorts of wens, curing wry necks and hair-lips without blemish'.)

Before long, Read's extravagant claims had been brought to the notice of Queen Anne. The queen suffered from a chronic weakness of the eyes, and was liable to fall an easy victim to any quack who would undertake to cure her of her infirmity. Read managed, somehow to persuade her that the treatments he prescribed were doing her good, and in 1705 the grateful woman, carefully made aware of the fact that he had also treated great numbers of her seamen and soldiers for blindness, gratis, gave him a knighthood and appointed him her Oculist-in-Ordinary.

Read's path to fame and fortune was then clear. In the following year, he published *A short but exact Account of all the Diseases incidental to the Eyes*, the latter part of which dealt in glowing terms with Read's various 'cures'. In this work, he announced his invention of 'styptic water', which he proposed to substitute, in many cases, for the barbaric cauterizations of the eye which were then in vogue. By 1711, Read was mixing with, and entertaining, most of the great aristocratic and literary figures of the day. On 11 April of that year, Dean Swift wrote to Stella:

> ... Henley would fain engage me to go with Steele, Rowe, Etc, to an invitation at Sir William Read's; surely you have heard of him; he has been a mountebank, and is the queen's oculist. He makes admirable punch, and treats you in golden vessels ...

After Read died in 1715 his widow, Lady Read, attempted to continue his business from the handsome house they had acquired in Durham Yard.

The position of London's Top Quack did not remain vacant for long.

A little later in the century, it was held very profitably by a man named Joshua Ward. Ward was born in 1685. He started his career with his brother in premises in Thames Street, where they carried on a business as drysalters.

This soon proved insufficiently exciting and glamorous for Ward, so, in 1717, he stood for parliament as the member for Marlborough and was duly elected. His success was quickly followed by a dispute about the propriety of his election. A committee was appointed to enquire into the affair. The members found that Ward had not, in fact, received a single vote, and he was unseated. After some more unsavoury political adventures he was forced to fly to France.

At that point in this short account of Ward's colourful career, it is appropriate to quote a paragraph from a rare pamphlet called *Physical Enquiries*, which was written by John Tennent and published in 1742:

> ... Joshua Ward Esq of Whitehall when in Paris became possessed of two *arcana*, which he styled his Pill and Drop, with which he practised Physic. There are many conjectures about his getting them, amongst which the most probable is that a Jesuit there communicated them to him; for as he had never studied physic, nobody can believe that he was the inventor of those secrets ...

The pill and drop that made Ward rich and famous are known, now, to have been composed principally of 'dragon's blood', or antimony, and wine. (His executors published the prescription, in 1763.) With one or both of his newly discovered remedies, Ward is said to have treated successfully a very sick Englishman who was living in Paris. Then—and in consequence of this unusual therapeutic feat—Ward managed to obtain, through the influence of his friend John Page, who was a member of parliament, a free pardon from King George II which allowed him to return to London. Established once more in the English capital, Ward started to advertise his nostrums, sending 'puffers' to go about the city into coffee houses and elsewhere to cry up to the skies the miraculous cures for which, he said, they had been responsible. Within a very few months, Ward's wares were the talk of the town. London's properly qualified physicians and apothecaries vehemently condemned Ward's 'absurd practice', saying that a person ignorant of physical learning who indiscriminately prescribed medicines of such a forcible nature as the pill and the drop would undoubtedly kill many of his misguided patients.

In spite of all the opposition he encountered, Ward eventually got a chance to treat the king himself.

His opportunity came when His Majesty was troubled by a violent pain in his thumb, which none of the officially appointed physicians and surgeons were able to relieve. Summoned to the royal residence, Ward took with him one of his infallible nostrums, which he concealed carefully in the palm of his hand. On being ushered with all due ceremony into the royal presence, Ward asked the king's permission to examine, closely, the painful thumb. Then, suddenly and unexpectedly, the quack gave the troublesome member so violent a wrench that the king cursed him, and kicked his shins, Ward bore this without complaint, and, when the king had cooled down, he respectfully asked his royal patient to move his thumb. The king did this easily, and found all his pain gone.

Nothing succeeds, in the quack world, like success. From that moment on, Ward's remedies were regarded with official favour—they became so respectable, in fact, that in 1753 the doctor's expensive fever powders were ordered for all ships in the British Navy—twenty-five powders being allowed for each vessel in the Channel Fleet, seventy-five for each vessel in the West Indies Station. The long-suffering British sailors continued to die in droves, in agony, as they had before.

William Hogarth—painter, engraver, and merciless scourge of all charlatans, in whatsoever walk of life they chose to operate—seized with glee on the misguided patronage given to Ward, and most cruelly depicted the 'pill and drop man' in his popular plate *The Undertaker's Arms or Consultation of Physicians*. Accompanying Ward, in this slashing attack on the quacks, Hogarth showed two other famous practitioners of the time—the 'Chevalier' Taylor, the roving oculist, and the huge and unprepossessing Sally Mapp.

Taylor had actually worked with William Cheselden at St

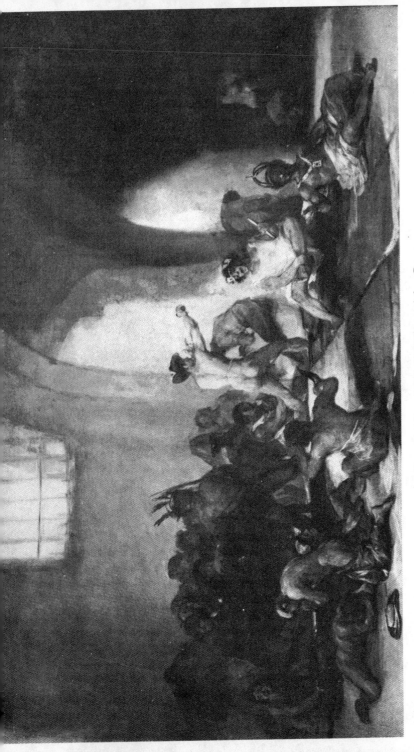

La Casa Dei Pazzi (The Madhouse) by Goya.

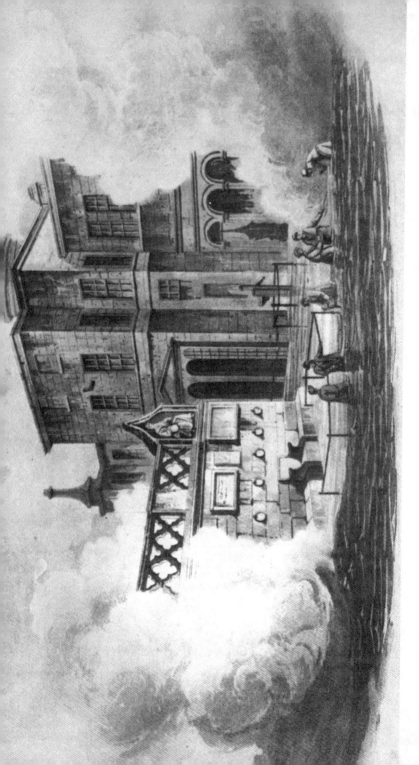

Taking the Waters, Bath, from an engraving by J. C. Nattes, 1806.

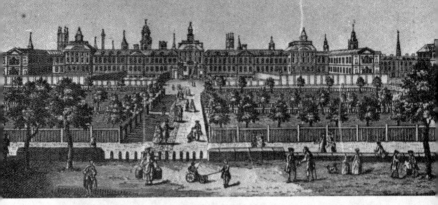

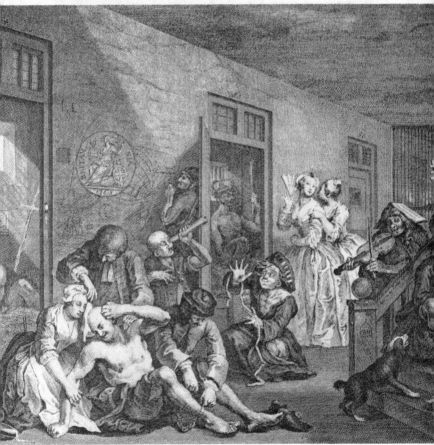

Top A view of the Hospital of Bethlehem after 1733, with additional wings for incurable patients. *Bottom A Rake's Progress* by Hogarth 1735 (plate VIII). Tom Rakewell's life of excesses has finally driven him completely mad, and he is chained up in Bedlam (Bethlehem Hospital)

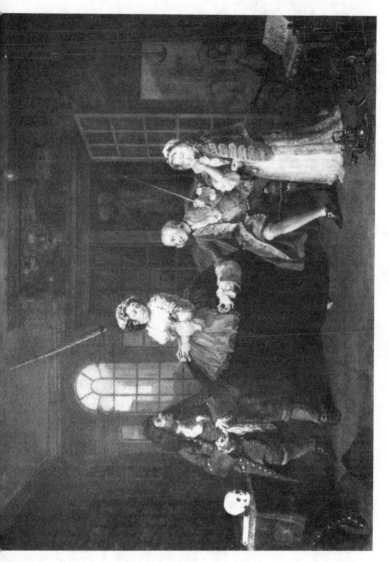

Marriage à la Mode by Hogarth 1745 (plate III). The Visit to the Quack. Viscount Squanderfield pays the price of his excesses, and imagines that the Quack has a form of medical knowledge which will help him.

Thomas's Hospital, so his claims to be an eye surgeon of some kind were not entirely bogus. It was Taylor's style of approach to the public that earned him Hogarth's ridicule—the Chevalier went round in black, wearing a long flowing wig, lecturing in a language remotely resembling Latin which the speaker described confidently but inaccurately as 'The True Ciceronian'. Among his patients, Taylor numbered Edward Gibbon, the historian, and Handel the composer, but his affected erudition did not impress Doctor Samuel Johnson, who said of him 'Taylor was the most ignorant man I ever knew, but sprightly'.

Sally Mapp—called frequently 'Crazy Sally'—was the daughter of a bone-setter who lived in a remote village in the county of Wiltshire.

Bone-setting, at that time, was a job that would normally be carried out, in a country district, by a farrier or 'vet'. It was not regarded, there, as a task that needed the expensive skills of a professional surgeon. The knack of setting bones successfully was commonly believed, in rural areas, to be transmitted hereditarily from father to son—or, in this single instance, from father to daughter. So 'Crazy Sally' grew up happily in her father's trade. Being, as it turned out, unusually competent or unusually lucky, Sally soon tired of a quiet country existence, and, leaving her pastoral home, she started to wander further afield. She settled, eventually, at Epsom, in Surrey, where her rare skills, and strength, earned her, in August 1736, this favourable notice in the *Gentleman's Review*:

> . . . The Cures performed by the Woman Bonesetter of *Epsom* are too many too be enumerated: Her bandages are extraordinarily Neat, and her Dexterity in reducing Dislocations and setting of fractured Bones wonderful. She has cured Persons who have been above 20 Years disabled, and has given incredible Relief in the most difficult Cases. The Lame came daily to her, and she got a great deal of Money, Persons of Quality who attended her Operations making her Presents . . .

Soon 'Crazy Sally' extended her practice to include a number of London cases. She performed some astonishing cures at the Grecian Coffee House, part of which she used, on her weekly visits to the capital, as an improvised consulting room. A few of her most spectacular feats were witnessed by the Grand Old Man of British Science, Sir Hans Sloane, who saw 'Crazy Sally' put right:

> ... A Man of *Wardour-Street* whose Back had been broke 9 Years, and stuck out 2 inches; a Niece of Sir *Hans Sloane* in the like Condition; and a Gentleman who went with one Shoe heel 6 inches high, having been lame 20 years, of his Hip and Knee; whom she set straight and brought his Leg down even with the other ...

As 'Crazy Sally' grew richer, her thoughts turned towards matrimony. She set her cap at one Hill Mapp, who was footman to a mercer in Ludgate Hill, reported the *Gentleman's Review*. The marriage was not successful—possibly, because the bride's strength was so great that she could reduce a dislocated shoulder without needing any assistance. Within a week of the wedding, the bridegroom had disappeared, taking with him one hundred guineas belonging to his hefty wife, and some of her portable property.

On her journeys between Epsom and London, Mrs Mapp drove in a splendid chariot drawn by four horses, and was accompanied by footmen and outriders clad in the richest liveries. On one of these journeys, when she was travelling along the Old Kent Road, she was mistaken by some pedestrians for an unpopular visitor from Europe. Her carriage was quickly surrounded by a hostile crowd. This was how the *Gentleman's Review* reported the incident:

> ... A Lady passing Kent-Street in her Chariot towards the Borough, dress'd in a Robe de Chambre, the People gave out she was a certain Woman of Quality from an Electorate in *Germany*, whereupon a great Mob follow'd and bestow'd on her many bitter Reproaches, till Madam perceiving some Mistake, look'd out and accosted them in this familiar Manner, *D—n your Bloods, don't you know me! I am Mrs Mapp the Bone-Setter.* Upon which they suddenly chang'd their Revilings into loud Huzza's ...

Soon after this, Mrs Mapp became so busy and successful that she decided to leave Epsom and to move to London, where she took a large house in the fashionable Pall Mall. Acting, as well as she could, the part of a great lady, she gave a plate worth ten guineas to be run for at the races at Epsom, and she went to see the race run. The first heat was won by a mare called 'Mrs Mapp'. The bone-setter was so delighted that she gave the jockey a guinea and promised to give him ninety-nine more if he won the plate but unfortunately for him the four-legged Mrs Mapp was not as energetic as her two-legged namesake. Percival Pott, the famous surgeon at St Bartholomew's Hospital, was to recall with disapproval this stage of the bone-setter's career:

. . . Even the absurdities and impractibility of her own promises and engagements were by no means equal to the expectations and credulity of those who ran after her, that is, of all ranks and degrees of people from the lowest labourer up to those of the most exalted rank and station, several of whom not only did not hesitate to believe implicitly the most extravagant assertions of this ignorant, illiberal, drunken, female savage, but even solicited her company or at least seemed to enjoy her society . . .

In the *Gentleman's Magazine* of October 1732, it was reported that Mrs Mapp had been with Joshua Ward and the Chevalier Taylor to the Playhouse in Lincoln's Inn Fields, to see a comedy called *The Husband's Relief*. The auditorium of the theatre was packed with people, and the grossly fat, unbelievably ugly woman heard these verses sung from the stage:

You Surgeons of London, who puzzle your Pates,
To ride in your Coaches, and purchase Estates,
Give over, for Shame, for your Pride has a Fall,
And ye Doctress of Epsom has outdone you all.

In Physick, as well as in Fashions, we find,
The newest has always its Run with Mankind,
Forgot is the Bustle 'bout *Taylor* and *Ward*;
Now *Mapp's* all ye Cry, & her Fame's on Record.

> Dame Nature has giv'n her a Doctor's Degree,
> She gets all ye Patients and pockets the Fee;
> So if you don't instantly prove her a Cheat,
> She'll loll in her Chariot while you walk ye street . . .

An epigram published shortly afterwards suggests that—as one might expect—Mrs Mapp appreciated the words of this song more than did either of the colleagues who were listening to it with her:

> While Mapp to th' actors shew'd a kind regard,
> On one side *Taylor* sat, on t'other *Ward*;
> When their mock Persons of the Drama came,
> Both *Ward* and *Taylor* thought it hurt their fame;
> Wondered how *Mapp* cou'd in good Humour be—
> *Zoons*, crys the Manly Dame, it hurts not *me*;
> Quacks without Art may either blind or kill;
> But *Demonstration* shews that mine is Skill . . .

The 'manly dame's' end was an unhappy one. Courted by so many of 'the most exalted rank and station', Mrs Mapp increased her rate of drinking until she was scarcely, if ever, sober. Her grand friends and patients forsook her, and she sank into poverty. She died, at a relatively early age, in some miserable lodgings in a narrow squalid street near the Seven Dials.

Seven years after *The Husband's Relief* caused 'House Full' notices to be displayed outside the Lincoln's Inn Fields theatre, another energetic female caught the attention of the London crowds. This was a Mrs Stephens, who marketed her mysterious 'Medicine for the Stone', advising that those who took it would not need to undergo the dreaded 'cut'. After publishing a list of the patients she claimed to have cured with her medicine, Mrs Stephens offered to sell to the public for £5,000 the secret of its composition. A parliamentary commission was appointed to enquire into her claims and to report into the wisdom—or otherwise—of accepting her offer. After prolonged deliberations, the members of the commission issued a certificate to the effect that the secrets of the composition and of the methods of production of Mrs Stephens' medicine had been fully revealed. It was made, they said, of egg-shells and calcined snails, with a decoction of some herbs, alicant, soap and honey. The signatories—who included the Archbishop of Canterbury and Sir William Chesel-den—added that they were convinced of the 'utility, efficacy and dissolving power thereof'. Not every properly qualified medical observer was entirely persuaded.

Among the doubters was a Doctor Jurin, who had been appointed first physician to Mr Guy's Hospital when it opened in 1725. Doctor Jurin was, himself, a sufferer from 'the gravel'. In his *Account of the Effects of Soap-Lye, take internally, for the Stone*, first published in 1742, the doctor described how he had managed to allay his sufferings by taking strong purgatives. About Christmas 1740, however, he had become extremely ill, owing to the passage of a stone from the kidney to the bladder, and he had voided 'a small red stone of the size of a pea'. In spite of the agonies he was suffering, he had refused to take the 'vaunted quack remedies' of Mrs Stephens. Instead, after reading the *Experiments and Observations* of Doctor Stephen Hales, FRS, on the dissolving power of soap lees, he had resolved to take some, knowing the substance to contain both lime and potash in abundance. After taking, experimentally, the new treatment for a few months in gradually increasing doses, he had started to feel better; had voided a succession of small stones, which, he said, showed signs of the solvent power of the lime; and, a little later, had considered himself perfectly cured.

The treatment of the Stone by any other means but operative surgery has been, until comparatively recent years, of negligible value. Attempts made during the eighteenth century to dissolve stones by internal remedies or by the injection of chemical agents into the bladder were—according to modern authorities—invariably worthless.

In 1745 Doctor Jurin brought out a new and revised edition of his treatise. In it, he confessed that although the drastic medicine he had previously recommended had conferred much benefit on many people, he had had to give up its use, owing to the extreme difficulty of obtaining it, whenever it was needed, in a consistent strength. His readers were not to worry, though. He had arranged with an apothecary for a supply of a substitute which would be 'almost free from nauseous taste or smell'. He apologized for having to conceal the manner of its preparation, but he assured his readers that this secrecy was only for the public benefit. The new liquid was to be called 'Lixivium Lithontripticum', and, said the doctor, he took it daily himself.

In spite of Doctor Jurin's confidence, his Lixivium Lithontripticum was soon to figure in a large-scale row. When he was called in to attend Robert Walpole, Earl of Orford, in the latter part of 1744, the doctor said that he had good reason to suppose that the nobleman was suffering from a stone in the bladder. Then, acting in conjunction with Sir Edward Hulse, he dosed the earl liberally with his 'Lixivium'. Although several stones were passed by the sufferer, the patient died on 18 March 1745. John Ranby, who was serjeant-surgeon to the king, unkindly then named Jurin's strong medicine as the probable cause of death and published a long *Narrative* of the case in which he expressed his opinion without any professional reserve. Jurin and Hulse retaliated in an anonymous *Epistle*. The controversy, which could never be satisfactorily settled, kept all parties concerned arguing away busily for quite a number of years.

Of all the men and women who performed some extraordinary pirouette on the lunatic fringe of eighteenth-century medicine, none were better fitted to fill the limelight, for a few brief instants, than the sincere but misguided Franz Anton Mesmer and the notorious quack James Graham.

Franz Mesmer was born in May 1734 at Itznang, which was a small village near Lake Constance. As a young man, Mesmer studied theology and medicine at the University of Ingolstadt, in Germany, and in Vienna. By the time he had graduated, he had become fascinated with the subject of the influence that the planets may have upon man. The stars, he believed, could affect the health and general physical condition of human beings through the medium of a subtle and invisible fluid that flows throughout the universe. Then, while experimenting with a magnet, Mesmer became convinced that his own hands held a force similar to that exerted by the magnet, and comparable to that exerted by the stars. In his case, he felt sure, the force could be used for healing.

In 1775 Mesmer first used the term 'animal magnetism' to describe the force that was emanating from his body. During the next three years, he recorded a number of strikingly successful cures—many of them, significantly, being with hysterical or emotionally disturbed patients. Then, in 1778, the more conventional medical men practising in Vienna accused him of dabbling in magic. His private séances were investigated by one of Maria Theresa's 'commissions', and he was ordered to leave the country within twenty-four hours.

Thrown out of Austria, Mesmer went to Spa, in Belgium, and from there he made his way to Paris. Once he had become known in the French capital, he caused a sensation, earning large sums of money as well as fame by his 'hypnotic séances'. At these performances, he wore a lilac-coloured suit and created a suitable atmosphere by playing a harmonica. Having got his audience into a conveniently receptive condition, Mesmer would touch each of his patients with a wand and then would stare piercingly into the sufferer's eyes. If any patient responded by showing symptoms of crisis, he or she would be led off to a private room for personal treatment. The theatrical nature of Mesmer's séances was emphasized by the 'magnetic tubs' he provided. These impressive stage properties were fitted with iron 'conductors'—ostensibly, for carrying the demonstrator's 'animal magnetism' to the patients, who were required to stand round them in a ring, holding each other's hands.

In Paris, as in Vienna, Mesmer's material successes roused the envy of more orthodox medical men, and he was denounced as an impostor and a charlatan. Then, in 1784, as the fuss grew, the French Government appointed a commission of scientists and physicians to investigate his activities. Benjamin Franklin was a member of this commission, which found that though Mesmer had undoubtedly effected many spectacular cures, his success was not due to any 'animal magnetism', as he claimed, but to some physiological cause that could not, at that time, be identified. The report, as a whole, was critical of Mesmer, and the poor man was driven from another flourishing practice—this time, to a life of obscurity in Switzerland. It is unfortunate that Mesmer, who was undoubtedly sincere in his beliefs, did not live to see hypnosis become one of the beneficial therapies of medical practice.

Mesmer's book, *Mémoire sur la découverte du Magnétisme Animal*, in which he expounded his ideas, was published in Paris and

Geneva in 1779. In the following year, the star of James Graham first started to shine brilliantly on the London scene.

James Graham—called frequently the 'Emperor of Quacks'—was born in 1745 in the Cowgates district of Edinburgh. After receiving some kind of a medical training, he journeyed to America where he practised with great success in Philadelphia. Having the advantages of a pleasing personality and a polite address, said one observer, Graham was able to introduce himself into the 'first circles', where he made a lot of money. Another observer noticed that when Graham went out walking 'all the women turned round to look at him'. That would have helped.

By 1779 Graham was back in Europe. After spending a short time as an oculist in the fashionable spa town of Bath, he moved to London, where he established himself in a fine house in the Royal Terrace in the Adelphi. In this elegant establishment, designed by the brothers Adam and furnished almost without heed to the expense, he established his Grand Temple of Health and of Hymen. Almost before Graham had had a chance to open the place, most of the grand folk in the capital, intrigued by his advertisements, were flocking to see it.

We know, from contemporary sources, more or less exactly what Graham's Temple was like. We know, for instance, that the house had an enormous golden star fixed on its front, and the words TEMPLUM AESCULAPIO SACRUM emblazoned over the entrance. Harry Angelo, who was court fencing-master to King George IV, included in his *Reminiscences* an eye-witness account of people arriving at the Temple for an evening performance:

> . . . I remember the carriages drawing up next to the door of this modern Paphos, with crowds of gaping sparks on either side, to discover who were the visitors, but the ladies' faces were covered, all going incognito. At the door stood two gigantic porters, each with a long staff, with ornamental silver head, like those borne by parish beadles, and wearing superb liveries, with large, gold-laced cocked hats, each was near seven feet high, and retained to keep the entrance clear . . .

One step took the visitor across the Adelphi's narrow pavement and into the Temple's entrance hall, where he or she would be relieved of an entrance fee of two guineas—in those days, a considerable sum. That paid, the visitor could begin the grand tour of the premises.

On the ground floor of the Temple was the central hall, which, like all the other rooms, was furnished lavishly, the walls being adorned with long draped mirrors. The spaces between the mirrors in the hall were occupied by offerings such as crutches, ear trumpets and other appliances that were said to have been left behind by grateful visitors who did not need them any more.

In the basement below the central hall was Graham's 'laboratory'—a workshop in which the doctor and his assistants prepared and sold his 'celebrated nostrums', which included an 'Electrical Aether', an 'Elixir of Life', 'Nervous Aetherial', and 'Imperial Pills'. In the first room above was Graham's 'cabinet', in which he sat to receive visitors who sought personal consultations.

Close by the 'cabinet' was the most lavishly appointed room of all—the 'Great Apollo Apartment', in which stood the 'Temple Sacred to Health'. In this room, on special occasions, an 'Ode set to Music' was performed by a 'selected choir', accompanied by an organ and a band of instrumentalists. Here, too, in the evenings, Graham delivered lectures—charging five shillings or half a crown extra for admission—and displayed his medico-electrical apparatus which included a 'Magnetic Throne' on which patients were required to sit if they were thought, by Graham, to need electrical treatment.

To illustrate his lectures, the proprietor of the Grand Temple used a series of attractive girls, who were referred to as Goddesses of Youth and Health. These girls—one of whom is said to have been Emma Hart, or Emma Lyons, who afterwards became Lady Hamilton—were required to pose in front of the audience in various degrees of undress. When Graham needed a new Goddess, he advertised like this:

> . . . Wanted genteel, decent, modest young woman; she must be personally agreeable, blooming, healthy, and sweet tempered and well recommended for modesty, good sense and steadiness. She is to live in the Physician's family, to be daily dressed in white silk robes with a rich rose coloured girdle. If

she can sing, play on the harpsichord or speak French greater wages will be given. Enquire Dr Graham, Adelphi Temple . . .

Attractive as the Goddesses may have been, their drawing power could hardly have been greater than Graham's supreme brain-child, the Grand Celestial Bed. This magnificent piece of apparatus was installed in a separate room that could be approached from the street by means of a private entrance—an understandable arrangement, when one considers what the bed was intended for. This is Graham's own description of the bed:

. . . The Grand Celestial Bed, whose magical influences are now celebrated from pole to pole and from the rising to the setting of the sun, is 12 ft long by 9 ft wide, supported by forty pillars of brilliant glass of the most exquisite workmanship, in richly variegated colours. The super-celestial dome of the bed, which contains the odoriferous, balmy and ethereal spices, odours and essences, which is the grand reservoir of those reviving invigorating influences which are exhaled by the breath of the music and by the exhilarating force of electrical fire, is covered on the other side with brilliant panes of looking-glass.

On the utmost summit of the dome are placed two exquisite figures of Cupid and Psyche, with a figure of Hymen behind, with his torch flaming with electrical fire in one hand and with the other, supporting a celestial crown, sparkling over a pair of living turtle doves, on a little bed of roses.

The other elegant group of figures which sport on the top of the dome, having each of them musical instruments in their hands, which by the most expensive mechanism, breathe forth sound corresponding to their instruments, flutes, guitars, violins, clarinets, trumpets, horns, oboes, kettledrums, etc.

The post or pillars too, which support the grand dome are groups of musical instruments, golden pipes, etc, which in sweet concert breathe forth celestial sounds, lulling the visions of Elysian joys.

At the head of the bed appears sparkling with electrical fire a great first commandment: 'BE FRUITFUL, MULTIPLY AND REPLENISH THE EARTH'. Under that is an elegant sweet-toned organ in front of which is a fine landscape of moving figures, priest and bride's procession entering the Temple of Hymen.

In the Celestial Bed no feather bed is employed but sometimes mattresses filled with sweet new wheat or oat straw mingled with balm, rose leaves, lavender flowers and oriental spices. The sheets are of the richest and softest silk, stained of various colours suited to the complexion. Pale green, rose colour, sky blue, white and purple, and are sweetly perfumed in oriental manner with the tudor rose, or with rich gums and balsams.

The chief principle of my Celestial Bed is produced by artificial lodestones. About 15 cwt of compound magnets are continually pouring forth in an everflowing circle.

The bed is constructed with a double frame, which moves on an axis or pivot and can be converted into an inclined plane.

Sometimes the mattresses are filled with the strongest, most springy hair, produced at vast expense from the tails of English stallions which are elastic to the highest degree . . .

In case anyone failed to understand exactly what the great bed was for, Graham used to explain in one of his lectures:

. . . Should pregnancy at any time not happily ensue, I have the most astonishing method to recommend which will infallibly produce a genial and happy issue, I mean my Celestial or Magnetico-electrico bed, which is the first and only ever in the world: it is placed in a spacious room to the right of my orchestra . . . Any gentleman and his lady desirous of progeny, and wishing to spend an evening in the Celestial apartment, after coition may, by a complement of a £50 bank note be permitted to partake of the heavenly joys it affords by causing immediate conception, accompanied by the soft music. Superior ecstacy which the parties enjoy in the Celestial Bed is really astonishing and never before thought of in this world: the barren must certainly become fruitful when they are powerfully agitated in the delights of love . . .

The 'agitation' and 'tilting' of the Grand Celestial Structure, cunningly devised by Graham and the ingenious engineer he employed, were clearly intended to help the impregnation of the ovum of one occupant of the bed by the spermatozoa of the other. The cost of a night in the bed—though given by Graham as £50—seems to have been increased under certain circumstances, as Angelo mentions in his *Reminiscences* that 'many a nobleman paid Graham £500 to draw the curtains'. Horace Walpole did not think that the performance was funny at all. He said that Graham's display was 'the most impudent puppet show of imposition' he had ever seen.

In 1781 Graham, encouraged by his success, took the larger and more imposing Schomberg House in Pall Mall. He fitted this place up at considerable expense and opened it as the 'Temple of Health and of Hymen'. His new establishment contained another 'Celestial State Bed' of greater magnificence even than the one that had been agitated and tilted in the Adelphi. At first, the crowds rolled up to Graham's new Temple, but within a very short time, in spite of all his flamboyant advertisements, posters and pamphlets, the enterprise started to fail. By 1783 Graham's creditors were pressing him for money. In a vain attempt to increase his income, Graham decided to lower his prices—always a dangerous expedient for a quack, when the demand for his wares is dropping. Fewer and fewer people went to Schomberg House, and soon Graham sold up, the Celestial State Bed being regarded as a realizable asset.

Graham's life, after that, was a sad decline from splendour. As soon as he could, he left London and started to wander through the provinces, giving lectures which on at least one occasion got him into trouble with the authorities. On his return to London, he attempted to found a new religious sect—a 'New and True Christian Church'—but this met with little support. The poet Southey said of him 'Graham was half-mad and his madness at last got the better of his knavery. He would madden himself with ether, run out into the streets, and strip himself to clothe the first beggar he met.' There is little doubt that Graham's mind did eventually become unhinged. He died suddenly at Edinburgh, at the age of forty-nine, in the year 1794.

During the whole of the eighteenth century, tuberculosis of the lungs—often called, for convenience, 'consumption'—was one of the most prevalent and most dreaded diseases on the American continent. As early as 1711 advertisements were appearing in America which claimed that a Mrs Masters' 'Tuscarora Rice' could effect an infallible cure for the lung rot. By 1733 the *New York Weekly Journal* was printing abstracts taken from the patents granted by His Majesty King George (who lived and ruled on the other side of the Atlantic) for 'Doctor Bateman's Pectoral Drops', which were said to be more effective, even, than Mrs Masters' Rice. In New York Province, King George's patents decreed, Doctor Bateman's drops were to be sold by one James Wallace, and by nobody else. A ten-guineas award was offered to anybody who could discover any person that counterfeited Doctor Bateman's medicine, or who sold such a counterfeit.

In that kind of climate, in which opportunities to get rich quickly were to be seized and protected from pirates and predators, purveyors of 'patent' or 'proprietary' medicines thrived. They relied, usually, on the press for reaching their potential customers, paying quite large sums for the insertion of lurid advertisements in national or local newspapers. In return for the badly needed revenue they provided, the newspapers' proprietors would usually insert, gratis, a few news items of the 'saved-from-a-horrible-death-by-Mr X's-pills' type. It was an arrangement that suited both the interested parties.

On 17 February 1796, the United States Patent Office, which had only been open for business for six years, had to consider an application from a Doctor Elisha Perkins.

Doctor Perkins was a properly qualified physician who had a flourishing practice in Windham County. He was one of the founder-members of the Connecticut Medical Society. He had done a certain amount of surgery and while he had been carrying out some operations he had noticed that when his metal instruments came into contact with certain of the patients' muscles, the muscles appeared to contract. Surely, he thought, he was generating some of the 'animal electricity' that had been described, over in Europe, by the clever professor Luigi Galvani? Surely, if he were, he could make some profitable use of this? He appeared before the Commissioner of Patents, and was granted a licence that allowed him, for seventeen years, the exclusive right to manufacture what he called his 'Metallic Tractors'.

Doctor Perkins' Metallic Tractors were made and sold in pairs.

Each pair consisted of two metal rods, about three inches long, which were made of brass and iron. Each rod was flattened on one side, and half round on the other. One of the rods' ends would be rounded; the other would be brought to a point. Doctor Perkins intended that the patient who bought a pair of the rods should 'draw' the disease from his or her body by rubbing the affected part with the two tractors, turn and turn about.

Months before he applied for a patent for his galvanic rods, Doctor Perkins told his colleagues in the Connecticut Medical Society of his great venture. Much to his surprise, he received very little encouragement from them. Undeterred by his fellow-members' lack of enthusiasm, the doctor took sample sets of the tractors to Philadelphia, where he gave some persuasive demonstrations with them in the public hospitals. Word went round that a miraculous new therapeutic device had appeared on the medical scene. Several members of Congress asked to be given the fullest possible information about the discovery, and Chief Justice Ellsworth was so impressed that he gave Doctor Perkins a letter of introduction to the incoming justice John Marshall. According to some reports, George Washington purchased a set of the tractors. Within a very few weeks, the invention was being talked of all over America. The doctor, working desperately hard at a small foundry 'concealed within a wall of his house', could hardly turn out enough of the little rods to satisfy the enormous demand.

Being a little envious, possibly, of the lucky inventor's financial success, the doctor's colleagues were less than happy about his unusual activities, and they advised him, soon, to close down his thriving business. The doctor disregarded their warnings, though, and he continued to make and sell his tractors. By 1797 he had become so unpopular with his fellows that he was expelled from membership of the Medical Society on the grounds that he was 'a patentee and user of nostrums'. Doctor Perkins—to use a modern platitude—cried all the way to the Bank.

As the craze for tractorization, in America, reached its peak, Perkins sent his son Benjamin Douglas across the Atlantic to open an office and saleroom in London. The tractors became, quickly, as well known and as easy to market in Britain as they were in America. They were given an entirely bogus air of respectability, in the Old World, by the foundation of a 'Perkinean Institution'.

This unreal and pretentious establishment had as its president a Right Honourable Lord Rivers and, as its vice-president, a Sir William Barker. In spite of this gratuitous 'puff' from these members of England's aristocracy, the sales appeal of Doctor Perkins' tractors faded rapidly in Britain, and the young man was soon forced to return, in some embarrassment, to the United States.

While he had been away, Father Perkins—alarmed at the rapidly falling sales of his tractors on their native heath—had been trying to market another startling remedy. This time, he had been offering a cure for the dreaded yellow fever. His new source of income was easier to make than any metallic rod—it was a simple mixture of common vinegar and muriate of soda. Quite confident of the efficacy of his second offering to suffering mankind, and eager to demonstrate its worth, Perkins took some to New York during a particularly virulent outbreak of the fever. The soda-vinegar medicine was shown, there, to be entirely and utterly useless. Perkins Senior caught the fever and within a few days he was dead.

In one instance, at least, the eighteenth-century quacks may be said to have outstripped and out-manoeuvred the professionals. That was, in the treatment of scabies, or 'the Itch'.

Augustus Hirsch, writing in 1885 on *Chronic Infective, Toxic, Parasitic, Septic and Constitutional Diseases*, said that among the parasitic diseases that had been known in every age and all parts of the world, the Itch took the foremost place. At one time, as many as 44.14 per cent of the inhabitants of Shanghai had been known to be suffering from the disease. Another writer, referring to the incidence of the trouble in Lower Brittany, said:

> . . . Scabies infests the individual several days after his birth, follows him throughout his entire life, and does not leave him until after his death . . .

We know, now, that scabies is caused by a tiny parasite—the *Acarus Scabiei*—which tunnels into human flesh.

The egg-bearing female starts just after her last moult to form the burrows in which she is going to lay her eggs. First, she gets a good grip on the skin by means of suckers on her front legs. Then, by propping up her body with the bristles on her back legs, she assumes an almost perpendicular position and begins cutting the skin. She does not take long to bore the first part of the tunnel—within two and a half minutes she may be completely concealed. Her pace, after that, depends largely on the warmth of her host's body. At a low temperature, or when the body of her host is cold, she is liable to cease burrowing altogether, but she is sure to start again on a slight rise in temperature or on a warming of the body. Normally, the parasite lives for four or five weeks in the burrow she has made, during which time she is likely to lay as many as two or three dozen eggs. The tiny creatures that hatch from these may then emerge, to repeat the uncomfortable cycle.

Quite early in the seventeenth century, the English writer Thomas Moffet appears to have realized that scabies is caused by a parasite:

> ... How cruel a disease this is, and to be compared with the lowsie disease, an honourable English Lady of sixty years knowes, she was the most vertuous Lady of *Penruddock* a knight, that by drinking too much Goats-milk (for she feared a consumption) was for ten years trouble with these wheal-worms, with which night and day she was miserably tortured in her eyes, lips, gums, soles of her feet, head, nose, and all her parts, that she lived a very grievous life, alwaies without rest, and at last in despite of all remedies, the disease increased, whereby her flesh was consumed, and she died thereof. I must not overpass this, that the more the women that sat by her, picked them out with their needles, the more their young ones bred, and when they had gnawed the flesh also, they grew to be bigger. Hence let proud despicable mankinde learn, that they are not only worms but worms-meat; and let us fear the power of that great God, who can with so contemptible an army counfound all pride, haughtiness, daintiness, and beauty, and conquer the greatest enemy ...

Cosimo Bonomo, in 1687, agreed with Moffet's tentative account of scabies and even prepared and published drawings of the horrific little parasite that caused the disease. Internal treatments—dosing with medicines and syrups, and the use of diuretics—

were quite useless, he said, and so was the blood-letting that was usually prescribed by all professors.

Bonomo's remarks were treated with derision by all properly qualified medical men. The disease was due to some 'disorder of the body humours', said the doctors, and they continued to draw blood merrily away from their tortured patients, and to pour into them such useless remedies as the compound of peppermint water, fennel water, corn-poppy blossoms and sulphuric acid that was recommended for the scabies-ridden troops throughout the Seven Years War. In all the history of medicine and surgery in the eighteenth century, no better illustration can be seen of the doctors' unfortunate habit of ignoring vital evidence and the correct explanation of facts, in favour of utterly false hypotheses. The truth, in this instance, should have been so ridiculously easy to verify, yet it was not verified, and hundreds of thousands of the doctors' misled patients itched on.

Sufferers who went to quacks for relief were—as suggested earlier—much more fortunate. Properly treated, scabies is readily curable, and almost by accident some 'gentlemen of experience'—and some ladies of their trade—seem to have stumbled on an effective remedy. One of these ease-giving women operated in colonial America, where the trouble was especially prevalent. In several issues of Benjamin Franklin's *Pennsylvania Gazette* in 1731 there appeared an advertisement inserted by Franklin's own mother-in-law, the Widow Read, who at the time was living at the home of her recently-married daughter and son-in-law:

... The Widow READ, removed from the upper End of Highstreet to the *New Printing Office* near the Market, continues to make and sell her well-known Ointment for the ITCH, with which she has cured abundance of People in and about this City for many Years past. It is always effectual for that purpose, and never fails to perform the Cure speedily. It also kills or drives away all Sorts of Lice in once or twice using. It has no offensive Smell, but rather a pleasant one; and may be used without the least Apprehension of Danger, even to a sucking Infant, being perfectly innocent and safe. Price 2s a Gallypot containing an Ounce; which is sufficient to remove the most inveterate Itch, and render the Skin clear and smooth ...

The exact composition of the Widow Read's ointment is not now known, but it is virtually certain that the contents of her gallypots —and the most successful anti-scabies salves sold by other quacks of the time—depended for their effectiveness on a high sulphur content.

The truth about scabies—suggested, again, by Johann Ernst Wichmann of Hamburg, in 1786—was not finally brought home to the members of the medical profession until 1834, when a doctor named Renucci, working in the skin clinic at the Hôpital St Louis in Paris, rediscovered the tiny creature that was entirely responsible for so much discomfort. Renucci's researches were of some importance in the history of medicine—for the first time ever, a definitely known cause had been established for one of the principal diseases of man. Long before bacteriologists and mycologists were in a position to throw proper doubt on Hippocrates's concept of the humours, Renucci, by his probings, had given the lie to some ancient, fallacious beliefs.

12

Medical and Surgical Support for the Armed Services in the Eighteenth Century

... Tweedledum and Tweedledee
Agreed to have a battle ...

CHARLES LUTWIDGE DODGSON
('LEWIS CARROLL'), 1832–98

It would be quite wrong to picture the typical eighteenth-century soldier as being anything like the sturdy, carefree godlike figure, dressed in a clean scarlet jacket and tight white buckskin breeches, who is featured in so many formal portraits painted at the time. It would be far more probable that the warrior of our period would resemble the wretched creature described in the Journal kept by Doctor Albigence Waldo, surgeon of Colonel Prentice's Connecticut Regiment at Valley Forge:

> ... There comes a soldier—His bare feet are seen through his wornout shoes—his legs nearly naked from the tattered remains of an only pair of stockings—his breeches not sufficient to cover his Nakedness—his shirt hanging in strings—his hair dishevelled—his face meagre—his whole appearance pictures a person forsaken and discouraged. This poor fellow comes to the doctor and cries with an air of wretchedness and despair, 'I am sick, my feet lame, my legs are soar, my body covered with this tormenting Itch, my clothes are worn out;' and so on ...

The 'tormenting Itch' referred to in that account was almost certainly scabies. A lot has been written about bubonic plague, malaria, smallpox, typhoid, typhus and yellow fevers, and other epidemic fevers which, because of their high mortality rates, have affected the size and striking power of the various armed services of history. Because scabies has not usually been fatal, it has been largely ignored by professional historians. In the eighteenth century, though, the tiny mites that burrowed into the soldiers' and sailors' flesh were liable to cause as much widespread distress as any opposing regiment or, at sea, any hostile squadron.

We know, for instance, how prevalent scabies was when the armies of Frederick the Great were in the field, for Johann Ackermann, who was an army doctor during the Seven Years War (1756–63) reported that the Itch was one of the most troublesome diseases with which he had to deal. Often, half the soldiers of a regiment would be infected with it, he said, and would have to be kept in some kind of hospital. Ernst Gottfried Baldinger, who was also a doctor in Frederick the Great's army, recalled that he often saw scabietic soldiers whose bodies were so completely crust-covered that not even the neck, the region of the thyroid gland, the breast or the abdomen were spared. Sometimes, he wrote, the green crust covering the body was completely hairy, and looked like moss. Baldinger believed that this malignant type of scabies affected soldiers more than anyone else. It could hardly be found in the homes of the civil population, he said, but it spread epidemically in the field hospitals. He thought that it was caused by the bad odour of diseased persons in the hospitals, by the overcrowding of patients, by the physical weakness of the exhausted soldiers, by their lack of cleanliness, and by their suppressed perspiration. Hardly anybody in the army escaped from the evil of scabies, he said, 'neither officer, nor physician, nor surgeon', the scabies-bitten soldier regarding the numerous red pustules produced by the disease as a normal accompaniment of his life. Baldinger himself suffered from scabies for more than a year.

In 1776 an English translation of a book entitled *The Diseases Incident to Armies, with the Method of Cure, etc,* written by a Baron van Swieten, was published 'for the Use of Military and Naval Surgeons in America'. Van Swieten was conscious of the great damage done to the morale of the services by scabies, but he attributed the Itch's spread to the fluid contents of the pustules.

'When these pustules are broke by scratching, the water that issues communicates the disorder to the neighboring parts,' he wrote, missing the point entirely.

Soldiers and sailors were not much more likely to escape scabies at the end of the eighteenth century, for—according to the medical historian August Hirsch—the sufferers from the Itch in the French armies fighting in the Napoleonic Wars could be counted 'by the hundred thousand'. Boris Sokeloff, describing Napoleon's Italian campaign of 1796–7, wrote: 'Whole regiments of soldiers, the moment they were encamped for the night, threw off their knapsacks and scratched en masse. The officers suffered no less than the soldiers; their commander-in-chief was no exception, scratching himself with a vengeance until blood appeared.' Edward Jenner, invited in 1802 to vaccinate a regiment of soldiers, gladly accepted, but when he reached the barracks he found so many men affected by the Itch that he had to abandon the whole project.

Scabies-infested or not, soldiers and sailors have to face in the field, or on the open sea, more predictable hazards than mites, and, in the course of their adventures, are not unlikely to sustain horrible wounds. During the eighteenth century, injured servicemen had to survive, if they could, in the most agonizing circumstances.

For a graphic account of the treatment of the wounded in the earlier decades of the century we can turn to the writings of Dominique Anel, who was surgeon-major in the French army during part of the reign of King Louis xiv. Educated surgeons who could be persuaded to travel with armies were few at that time, he records, and their place was usually filled by unqualified persons who called themselves 'wound suckers'. Some of these 'suckers' were old soldiers; others had never seen any active service. All were entirely ignorant of surgery. They all pretended that they could cure wounds by sucking them, after which they would pour in a little oil, would mutter certain magic charms, and then would cover the whole with a compress. The charms, said Anel, were nonsense; the oil did neither harm nor good; the sucking was sometimes of great value because it could remove blood clots and foreign bodies that might prevent the flesh re-uniting. Anel, finding the operation dangerous and disgusting when done with the mouth, invented an ingenious suction syringe which would do the job automatically.

Another French army surgeon—Jean Louis Petit—found that his experiences in the field stimulated his inventive powers. In Petit's case, his greatest achievements were probably the development of the famous 'screw' tourniquet and the improvements he made to the circular method of amputation. Petit eventually became director of the French Royal Academy of Surgery, which was established in 1731 and which did a great deal to improve surgery and to raise the status of the surgeon in France.

Prior to the year 1775, there was no proper army in America and therefore there was no official Army Medical Department. The few colonial militia organizations—widely separated, without a common command, and modelled loosely on the style of English regiments—appointed local surgeons, such as they were and if they could be found, to attend to the needs of the men of all ranks who might become sick, or who might be wounded. Among the more unfortunate patients these men might be called upon to treat were those who had been scalped by Red Indians. James Thacher, MD, who served throughout the whole War of Independence as a surgeon's mate in hospital and as a regimental surgeon, wrote a *Military Journal* which is a valuable source of information about this and other hazards. Here is a revealing extract:

> . . . Captain Greg was immediately carried to the fort, where his wounds were dressed. He was afterwards removed to our hospital, and put under my care. He was a most frightful spectacle; the whole of his scalp was removed; in two places on the fore part of his head the tomahawk had penetrated through the skull; there was a wound on his back with the same instrument, besides a wound in his side and another through his arm by a musket ball. This unfortunate man, after suffering extremely for a long time, finally recovered, and appeared to be well satisfied in having his scalp restored to him, though uncovered with hair. The Indian mode of scalping their victims is this—with a knife they make a circular cut from the forehead quite round, just above the ears, then taking hold of the skin with their teeth, they tear off the whole hairy scalp in an instant, with wonderful dexterity . . .

Illuminating, too, is the *Journal of Isaac Senter, Physician and Surgeon of the Troops detached from the American Army encamped at Cambridge, Mass, on a secret Expedition against Quebec, under the command of Col. Benedict Arnold, in September 1775.* Senter's journal, published by the Historical Society of Pennsylvania in 1846, gives a grim picture of an ill-fated expedition undertaken with little advance planning, and launched in the face of almost insuperable difficulties. Half of the command of eleven hundred had had enough after six weeks, and turned back. The other half of the force pressed on through the desolate northern territories. As they marched, the men's inadequate rations of flour and partly-spoiled salt pork dwindled steadily until they were, at last, entirely without food and threatened with starvation. Those who were unable to keep going had to be left to die in the wilderness. Without tents or shelter, having lost all their camping equipment and most of their ammunition, the shrunken party won through snow and ice to Quebec, where they found that they had only four rounds of ammunition per man left for the attack. When the attack failed, the force managed to keep up a siege for some months in the face of great discouragement. General Montgomery was killed; Colonel Arnold wounded; General Thomas perished with smallpox. Senter had lost his instruments and medicines on the nightmare journey to Quebec, but he had managed to save a pocket lancet and was still able to indulge in as much ritual blood-letting as he wished. Pneumonia, pleurisy and smallpox he had to treat, perforce, without medicines, though he may have done this more successfully than he would have if his usual remedies had been to hand. After General Thomas's death, Senter carried out smallpox inoculation on a large scale, noting in his journal in May 1776:

> ... I generally inoculated a regiment at a class, who had it so favourable as to be able to do garrison duty during the whole time ...

In several other military exploits in the American War of Independence, a lack of proper preparation seems to have caused an enormous amount of human suffering. In his book *Gentleman Johnny Burgoyne*, published by the Bobbs-Merrill Company in 1927,

F J Hudleston suggested that General Gage may have made no provision at all for the men likely to be wounded at the battle of Bunker Hill. 'It did not occur to him that you can not make an omelet without breaking eggs and that a battle is necessarily attended by casualties,' commented Hudleston. An eye-witness described the scene in this way:

> . . . It is impossible to describe the horror that on every side presented itself—wounded and dead officers on every street; the town [Boston], which is larger than New York, almost uninhabited to appearance, bells tolling, wounded soldiers lying in their tents and crying for assistance to remove some men who had just expired. So little precaution did General Gage take to provide for the wounded by making hospitals, that they remained in this deplorable situation for three days; the wounded officers obliged to pay the most exorbitant price for lodgings . . .

In 1777 there was published, 'by order of the Board of War', a small pamphlet called *Directions for Preserving the Health of Soldiers* which had been compiled with misplaced optimism by Doctor Benjamin Rush of Pennsylvania. Among Doctor Rush's gems of wisdom the American army surgeons would have seen:

> . . . It is a well-known fact, that the perspiration of the body, by attaching itself to linen, and afterwards, by mixing with rain, is disposed to form miasmata, which produce fevers . . .

'By virtue of his social and professional prominence, his position as teacher and his facile pen,' the modern historian P M Ashburn has commented in his *History of the Medical Department of the United States Army*, 'Benjamin Rush had more influence upon American medicine and was more potent in the propagation and long perpetuation of medical errors than any man of his day. To him, more than to any other man in America, was due the great vogue of vomits, purging, and especially of bleeding, salivation and blistering, which blackened the record of medicine and afflicted the sick almost to the time of the Civil War.'

Throughout the eighteenth century, and for some time after, the wholesale surgery that had to follow a battle was a grim and bloody business. One of the most harrowing first-hand accounts comes from the diary of William Beaumont, pioneer physiologist, who was born at Lebanon, Connecticut, on 21 November 1785. Beaumont was present in September 1812 when the British were driven from their garrison in York Town and, on evacuating their stronghold, decided to blow up their magazine which contained, at the time, hundreds of barrels of gunpowder. The explosion that resulted almost totally destroyed the American force. More than three hundred American men were wounded, and about sixty were killed dead on the spot by stones of all sizes falling like a shower of hail in the midst of their ranks. Beaumont wrote in his diary:

... A most distressing scene ensues in the Hospital—nothing but the Groans of the wounded and agonies of the Dying are to be heard. The Surgeons wading in blood, cutting off arms, legs, and trepanning heads to rescue their fellow creatures from untimely deaths. To hear the poor creatures crying, 'Oh, Dear! Oh, Dear! Oh, my God, my God! Do, Doctor, Doctor! Do cut off my leg, my arm, my head, to relieve me from misery! I can't live, I can't live!' would have rent the heart of steel, and shocked the insensibility of the most hardened assassin and the cruelest savage. It awoke my liveliest sympathy, and I cut and slashed for 48 hours without food or sleep. My God! Who can think of the shocking scene when his fellow-creatures lie mashed and mangled in every part, with a leg, an arm, a head, or a body ground in pieces, without having his very heart pained with the acutest sensibility and his blood chill in his veins ...

After suspending his operations to take a little refreshment to sustain life ('the first time since four o'clock yesterday') Beaumont returned again to the 'bloody scene of distress':

... To continue dressing, Amputating and Trepanning. Dressed rising of 50 patients, from simple contusions to the worst of compound fractures, more than half of the last description. Performed two cases of amputation and one of trepanning. 12 Ock PM retired to rest my much fatigued body and mind . . .

One of the greatest of all military surgeons—Dominique Jean Larrey, afterwards Baron Larrey—was born in 1766 and served all through the Napoleonic Wars. During the winter of 1789, Larrey witnessed the street fighting that ushered in the French Revolution and a large number of the wounded came under his direct supervision in the Hôtel Dieu. Soon after that, France was at odds with the rest of Europe, and Larrey was appointed surgeon to the army of the Rhine. In the course of this campaign, Larrey originated the idea of First Aid to the wounded by designing, and having constructed, his ingenious 'Ambulances Volantes', or Flying Ambulances. Up to that time, it had been the customary practice to station the members of the surgical staff and their assistants at the rear of the troops, the injured being left on the battlefield until all the fighting was over. Larrey, without thinking of his own safety, preferred to dash into the thick of the fray with his novel vehicles, which were of two kinds—light, closed, two-wheeled carriages, drawn by two horses, that could make swift progress over relatively even ground; and heavier, slower, four-wheeled carts, drawn by four horses, which would accommodate four men and were more suitable for use in rough terrain. The ambulances were fitted with portable litters, or 'stretchers', and they carried splints, bandages, medicines and food. Larrey's new, humane aids justifiably caused a sensation and similar vehicles were soon ordered for use by all the armies of the Republic.

In 1794 Larrey met Napoleon Bonaparte at Toulon, and the two men became close friends. Larrey was present at no fewer than sixty battles and was wounded at least three times. When British forces attacked Alexandria in 1801, the great French surgeon had just finished amputating the thigh of the sixty-year-old General Silly, when he happened to notice that he had been deserted by all his assistants except one, and he was disturbed to see that a squadron of English cavalry was moving in a determined way towards his ambulance. Picking up the so-recently de-limbed general and placing him on his shoulders, Larrey ran for safety, choosing, to serve as his best route, a field that had been recently dug with holes for the cultivation of capers. The English cavalrymen, unable owing to the holes to take their horses over the ground in pursuit, had to watch the distinguished but incongruously adjusted pair of foreigners get unharmed away. Both Frenchmen reached Alexandria safely, and the general made a complete recovery from his extraordinary and uncomfortable experience.

At this distance of time, it would be difficult for anyone to decide whether eighteenth-century soldiers or eighteenth-century sailors had more difficulties and discomforts with which to contend. In his long and satirical novel *The Adventures of Roderick Random*, first published in 1748, Tobias Smollett painted a horrifying picture of the sufferings inflicted on sick sailors during the period with which he was dealing. There is a strong element of caricature in everything that ever came from Smollett's pen, but as he is known to have been writing from direct personal experience it is safe to assume that his descriptions were not entirely fanciful.

Smollett was a Scotsman who travelled in 1739 from his native Dumbartonshire to London in a vain attempt to win fame and fortune as a playwright. When no one of any consequence in the English capital would consider producing the only play he had written, he managed to get a post as a surgeon's mate on board a battleship in the squadron of Sir Chaloner Ogle, who was then about to sail to the West Indies to reinforce the fleet commanded by Admiral Edward Vernon. Roderick Random, in Smollett's picaresque story, contrives similarly to obtain employment afloat. So, this account of Random's qualifying visit to the Surgeons' Hall has at least a partial ring of truth:

. . . I preserved my half-guinea entire till the day of examination, when I went with a quaking heart to Surgeons' Hall, in order to undergo that ceremony. Among a crowd of young fellows who walked in the outward hall, I perceived Mr Jackson, to whom I immediately went up, and . . . asked what his business was in this place? He replied, he was resolved to have two strings to his bow, that in case the one failed he might use the other; and, with this view, he was to pass that night for a higher qualification. At that instant a young fellow came out from the place of examination with a pale countenance, his lip quivering, and his looks as wild as if he had seen a ghost. He no sooner appeared, than we all flocked about him with the utmost eagerness to know what reception he had met with; which, after some pause, he described, recounting all the questions they had asked, with the answers he made. In this manner we obliged no less than twelve to recapitulate, which, now the danger was past, they did with pleasure, before it fell to my lot . . .

At last, the beadle called Random's name, with a voice that made the young man tremble as much as if it had been the sound of the last trumpet:

. . . However, there was no remedy: I was conducted into a large hall, where I saw about a dozen of grim faces sitting at a long table; one of whom bade me come forward, in such an imperious tone that I was actually for a minute or two bereft of my senses. The first question he put to me was, 'Where was you born?' To which I answered, 'In Scotland.'—'In Scotland,' said he; 'I know that very well; we have scarce any other countrymen to examine here; you Scotchmen have overspread us of late as the locusts did Egypt: I ask you in what part of Scotland was you born?' I named the place of my nativity, which he had never before heard of: he then proceeded to interrogate me about my age, the town where I served my time, with the term of my apprenticeship; and when I informed him that I served three years only, he fell into a violent passion; swore it was a shame and a scandal to send such raw boys into the world as surgeons; that it was a great presumption in me, and an affront upon the English, to pretend to sufficient skill in my business, having served so short a time, when every apprentice in England was bound seven years at least; that my friends would have done better if they had made me a weaver or shoemaker, but their pride would have me a gentleman, he supposed, at any rate, and their poverty could not afford the necessary education . . .

This exordium did not at all contribute to the recovery of Random's spirits:

. . . But, on the contrary, reduced me to such a situation that I was scarce able to stand; which being perceived by a plump gentleman who sat opposite me, with a skull before him, he said, Mr Snarler was too severe upon the young man; and turning towards me, told me, I need not be afraid, for nobody would do me any harm; then bidding me take time to recollect myself, he examined me touching the operation of the trepan, and was very well satisfied with my answers. The next person who questioned me was a wag, who began by asking if I had ever seen amputation performed; and I replying in the affirmative, he shook his head, and said, 'What! upon a dead subject, I suppose?' 'If,' continued he, 'during an engagement at sea, a man should be brought to you with his head shot off, how would you behave?' After some hesitation, I owned such a case had never come under my observation, neither did I remember to have seen any method of cure proposed for such an accident, in any of the systems of surgery I had perused. Whether it was owing to the simplicity of my answer, or the archness of the question, I know not, but every member at the board deigned to smile, except Mr Snarler, who seemed to have very little of the *animal visibile* in his constitution. The facetious member, encouraged by the success of his last joke, went on thus: 'Suppose you was called to a patient of a ple-thoric habit, who had been bruised by a fall, what would you do?' I answered, I would bleed him immediately. 'What,' said he, 'before you had tied up his arm?' But this stroke of wit not answering his expectation, he desired me to advance to the gentleman who sat next to him; and who, with a pert air, asked what method of cure I would follow in wounds of the intestines. I repeated the method of cure as it is prescribed by the best chirurgical writers; which he heard to an end, and then said, with a supercilious smile, 'So you think by such treatment the patient might recover?'—I told him I saw nothing to make me think otherwise. 'That may be,' resumed he, 'I won't answer for your foresight; but did you ever know of a case of this kind succeed?' I answered I did not; and was about to tell him I had never seen a wounded intestine; but he stopped me, by saying, with some precipitation, 'Nor never will. I affirm, that all wounds of the intestines, whether great or small, are mortal.'—'Pardon me, brother,' says the fat gentleman, 'there is very good authority—' —Here he was interrupted by the other with 'Sir, excuse me, I despise all authority. *Nullius in verba.* I stand upon my own bottom.'—'But, sir, sir,' replied his antagonist, 'the reason of the thing shows—' —'A fig for reason,' cried this sufficient member, 'I laugh at reason, give me ocular demonstration.' The corpulent gentleman began to wax warm, and observed that no man acquainted with the anatomy of the parts would advance such an extravagant assertion. This innuendo enraged the other so much that he started up, and in a furious tone exclaimed, 'What, sir! do you question my knowledge in anatomy?' By this time, all the examiners had espoused the opinion of one or other of the disputants, and raised their voices all together, when the chairman commanded silence, and ordered me to withdraw. In less than a quarter of an hour I was called in again, received my qualification sealed up, and was ordered to pay five shillings . . .

When Roderick Random delivered his letters of qualification to the Navy Office, he was 'mightily pleased' to find himself thought suitable to be the surgeon's second mate on a third rate vessel. Having insufficient money to bribe the secretary, however, he was pushed out of the office without being offered a vacancy. While he was waiting vainly for a sea-going post—either on an existing ship, or on one that was to be soon put into commission—he was offered a job as a 'journeyman' or assistant to a French apothecary. According to Smollett, Random's temporary employer could:

. . . Make up a physician's prescription, though he had not in his shop one medicine mentioned in it. Oyster shells he could invent into crab's eyes; common oil into oil of sweet almonds; syrup of sugar, into balsamic syrup; Thames water, into aqua cinnamoni; turpentine, into capivi; and a hundred more costly preparations were produced in an instant, from the cheapest and coarsest drugs of the *materia medica*: and when any common thing was ordered for a patient, he always took care to disguise it in colour or taste, or both, in such a manner as that it could not possibly be known. For which purpose cochineal and oil of cloves were of great service . . .

Captured, before long, by a press gang and carried off to sea, Random found himself on a ship which had, as its surgeon, a 'good-natured indolent man'. After suffering some grave misadventures, Random was invited to serve this indolent person as his third mate, to supply the place of a man who had recently died. This appointment did not do much to raise the pressed man's status on shipboard, however, for the ship's captain was 'too much of a gentleman to know a surgeon's mate, even by sight'. (The ship's chaplain would have been treated with ignominy, too, being required to use the men's latrines or 'round house' in the bows rather than the officers' convenience near the stern of the ship.)

At seven o'clock in the evening, the surgeon's first mate visited the sick and ordered what was proper for each. The new third mate was then asked to assist the second mate in making up the prescriptions ordered by their superior colleague. When Random, carrying the medicines, followed his immediate senior into the sick berth or hospital, and observed the situations of the patients, he was understandably horrified:

> . . . I was much less surprised that people should die on board, than that any sick person should recover. Here I saw about fifty miserable distempered wretches, suspended in rows, so huddled one upon another, that not more than fourteen inches space was allotted for each with his bed and bedding; and deprived of the light of day, as well as of fresh air; breathing nothing but a noisome atmosphere of the morbid steams exhaling from their own excrements and diseased bodies, devoured with vermin hatched in the filth that surrounded them, and destitute of every convenience necessary for people in that helpless condition . . .

Random could not comprehend 'how it was possible for the attendants to come near those who hung on the inside towards the sides of the ship, in order to assist them, as they seemed barricadoed by those who lay on the outside, and entirely out of reach of all visitation'. He soon found out, though, when he saw the second mate, who was required to administer some clysters that had been ordered, 'thrust his wig in his pocket, and strip himself to his waistcoat in a moment, then creep on all-fours under the hammocks of the sick, and, forcing up his bare pate between two, keep them asunder with one shoulder, until he had done his duty.'

Attending to the wounded during and after a naval engagement during the eighteenth century must have been a harrowing business, since all would have to be done in surroundings as cramped and as crowded as that. Edward Ward, who was surgeon in Admiral Watson's flagship in the Indian Ocean in 1775, described his difficulties in a book that he called *Voyage from England to India*:

> ... At the very instant when I was amputating the limb of one of our wounded seamen, I met with an almost continual interruption from the rest of his companions, who were in the like distressed circumstances; some pouring forth the most piercing cries to be taken care of, while others seized my arm in their earnestness of being relieved, even at the time when I was passing the needle for securing the divided blood vessels by a ligature. Surely, at the time when such operations are in contemplation, the operator's mind as well as body ought to be as little agitated as possible; and the very shaking of the lower gun deck, owing to the recoil of the large cannon which are placed just over his head, is of itself sufficient to incommode a surgeon ...

The normal operating theatre was the 'cockpit'—a small ill-ventilated den situated on the orlop deck below the water line and illuminated only by lanterns. In an emergency, other places in the lower parts of the ship might have to be made available for the surgeon. Robert Young, surgeon in HMS *Ardent* at the battle of Camperdown in 1797 left, in his unpublished journal, now in the possession of the British Admiralty, an unforgettable picture of the aftermath of a naval engagement of the time. Young had no mate to assist him, since many of these had left the service after the recent naval mutinies:

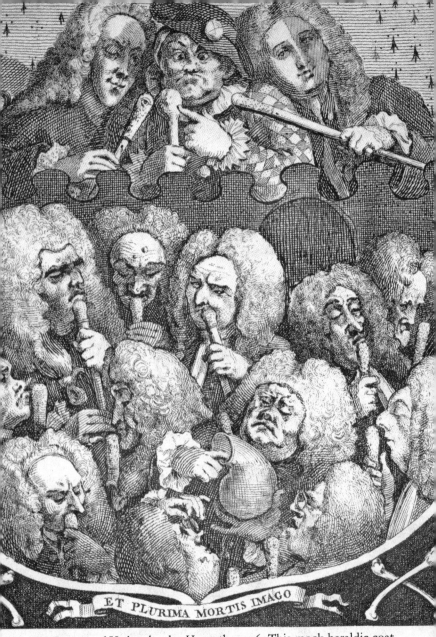

The Company of Undertakers by Hogarth, 1736. This mock heraldic coat of arms depicts many of the charlatans of the period. The three "doctors" at the top of the escutcheon are supposed to represent Sally Mapp, the Epsom bone setter, Joshua ("Spot") Ward, and John Taylor, a quack oculist.

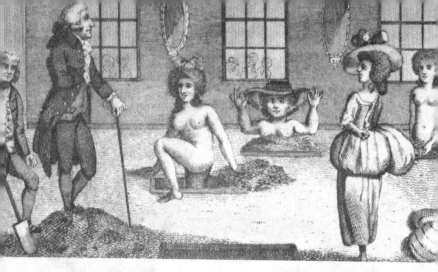

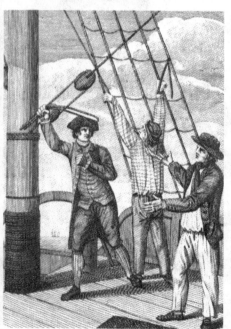

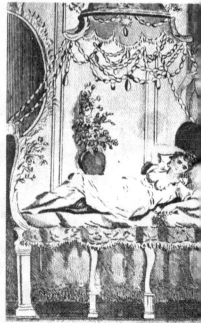

Top James Graham's Mud Bathes (Ramblers Magazine 1726?). This famous quack persuaded many ladies of quality that this was a new way of preserving health and beauty. *Lower left* Kenneth Hossack flogged and murdered by James Lowry, Captain of a Jamaica ship. Engraved for the Malefactors' Register. Newgate Calendar Volume III. *Lower right* James Graham's Grand Celestial Bed, situated in his Temple of Health and Hymen. He charged £50 or more per night to sleep in it, and claimed that the childless who did so would become prolific.

. . . I was employed in operating and dressing till near 4.0 in the morning, the action beginning about 1.0 in the afternoon. So great was my fatigue that I began several amputations under a dread of sinking before I should have secured the blood vessels.

Ninety wounded were brought down during the action. The whole cockpit deck, cabins, wing berths and part of the cable tier, together with my platform and my preparations for dressing were covered with them. So that for a time they were laid on each other at the foot of the ladder where they were brought down, and I was obliged to go on deck to the Commanding Officer to state the situation and apply for men to go down the main hatchway and move the foremost of the wounded further forward into the tiers and wings, and thus make room in the cockpit. Numbers, about sixteen, mortally wounded, died after they were brought down, amongst whom was the brave and worthy Captain Burgess, whose corpse could with difficulty be conveyed to the starboard wing berth. Joseph Bonheur had his right thigh taken off by a cannon shot close to the pelvis, so that it was impossible to apply a tourniquet; his right arm was also shot to pieces. The stump of the thigh, which was very fleshy, presented a dreadful and large surface of mangled flesh. In this state he lived near two hours, perfectly sensible and incessantly calling out in a strong voice to me to assist him. The bleeding from the femoral artery, although so high up, must have been very inconsiderable, and I observed it did not bleed as he lay. All the service I could render this unfortunate man was to put dressings over the part and give him drink.

In many other instances I had occasion to observe that vessels collapse and bleed little after gunshot or splinter wounds. The vessel probably stretched longitudinally has its sides brought more together, and the cavity diminished; when at length transversely separated by violence, the jagged ends detract inwards, which with the spasmodic contraction of the circular fibres of the artery, occasioned by the tension, completely closes the passage and resists the impetus of the blood from above. Whether this attempt to describe be just or not, the fact is deserving of notice.

Melancholy cries for assistance were addressed to me from every side by wounded and dying, and piteous moans and bewailing from pain and despair. In the midst of these agonising scenes, I was able to preserve myself firm and collected, and embracing in my mind the whole of the situation, to direct my attention where the greatest and most essential services could be performed. Some with wounds, bad indeed and painful, but slight in comparison with the dreadful condition of others, were most vociferous for my assistance. These I was obliged to reprimand with severity as their voices disturbed the last moments of the dying. I cheered and commended the patient fortitude of others, and sometimes extorted a smile of satisfaction from the mangled sufferers, and succeeded to throw momentary gleams of cheerfulness amidst so many horrors. The man whose leg I had first amputated had not uttered a groan from the time he was brought down, and several, exulting in the news of the victory, declared they regretted not the loss of their limbs . . .

A man who was at once physician, surgeon and apothecary, upon whom the health and lives of so great a number of valuable subjects of the State were often solely depending, ought to have every means and every instrument and every accommodation to favour and aid the exercise of his industry and skill, said the man who had sometimes extorted a smile of satisfaction from the mangled sufferers. But such necessary benefits lay in the far distant future. For making up and keeping at hand a 'regular formula of extemporaneous medicines', for having everything he might want ready of access—his instruments, lint, needles, his lotions, dressings, pills, etc.—Young had 'no convenience whatever'. The expense of providing a 'well contrived Dispensatory', he was sure, 'would be trivial'. Trivial or not, this was a luxury that their Lordships of the Admiralty were not able, or willing, at that precise moment in history, to afford.

The diseases most feared by those serving on board ship during the eighteenth century were fevers, 'fluxes' (illnesses, such as dysentery, that involved some morbid or excessive discharge of blood or excrement, or both), and scurvy.

One of the most disastrous outbreaks of scurvy ever experienced marred Commodore Anson's voyage round the world in 1740–44. In order to fill his flagship *Centurion*, and five other ships which were to accompany him, Anson was offered 350 seamen. Of these, only 175 reported on board, thirty-two of these men having been discharged, immediately before, from the Haslar Hospital near Portsmouth. Anson had hoped to take with him a whole able-bodied marine regiment. Instead of these active young men, he was given a draft of five hundred invalids from the out-pensioners of London's Chelsea Hospital—men who from their age and disabilities were regarded as unfit for service in a marching regiment. The Commodore, according to his chaplain, 'was greatly chagrined at having such a decrepit detachment allotted to him.' But only 259 reached Anson, 'for all those who had limbs and strength enough to walk out of Portsmouth deserted, leaving behind them only such as were literally invalids, most of them being sixty years of age, and some upwards of seventy.'

The ships left the south coast of England at an unfavourable time of the year. By the time they reached the Pacific, the provisions were mouldy and most of the men were suffering from the dreaded scurvy:

... The disease extended itself so prodigiously [reported the Commodore's chaplain] that after the loss of over 200 men we could not, at last, muster more than six foremast men in a watch capable of duty ...

The symptoms of scurvy were inconstant and innumerable, recorded the chaplain, scarcely any two persons ever being found to be suffering in the same way. There were, however, some symptoms more general than the rest which, he thought, deserved particular mention. These included:

... Large discoloured spots, dispersed upon the whole surface of the body, swelled legs, putrid gums, and above all, an extraordinary lassitude of the whole body, especially after any exercise, however inconsiderable; and this lassitude, at last degenerates into a proneness to swoon, and even die, on the least exertion of strength, or even on the least motion. This disease is likewise attended with a strange degeneration of spirits, with shiverings, tremblings, and a disposition to be seized with the most dreadful terrors on the slightest accident ...

Other misfortunes suffered by the scurvy patients on the *Centurion* included jaundice, pleurisy, and the outbreak of ulcers forming 'a luxuriancy of fungous flesh'—the sailors called these ulcers 'bullock's liver'. Old and healed wounds tended to reopen, too. One veteran who had fought at the Battle of the Boyne fifty years before died from the reopening of an injury he had sustained there.

The only remedy for scurvy carried on board Anson's ships, as far as can be established, was 'elixir of vitriol'—compounded of oil of vitriol, spirits of wine, sugar, cinnamon, ginger and other spices—which had been recommended by the College of Physicians and approved by Admiral Vernon. The elixir was just about as effective as Doctor 'Spot' Ward's famous pill and drop, described in Chapter 9. Of the 510 men who had left England on the *Centurion*, only 130 returned home.

Three years after they got back, Doctor John Huxham, of Totnes in Devon, recommended that 1200 sailors of Admiral Martin's fleet who had been disabled by scurvy should be put on a vegetable diet. The long, hopeless battle against this crippling disease was at last in sight of being won.

13

Old Age in the Eighteenth Century, and Death—The Last Enemy in all Periods of History

... Do not ask for whom the bell tolls;
It tolls for Thee ...

JOHN DONNE, ?1571–1631

Anyone who has read the preceding chapters of this book will know how difficult it was for any European or American person in the eighteenth century to stay alive. The number of people who managed to survive the pains and perils of infancy, youth and middle age was not, therefore, great—certainly, there were far fewer 'senior citizens' to be seen around then, in relation to the population as a whole, than there are today, and those that did manage to go on existing beyond man's allotted span of three score years and ten were regarded as quite remarkable. A report in the *Gentleman's Magazine* of November 1732 suggests that the behaviour of these veterans was sometimes a little trying:

... It is from the implicit Respect, to which old Men lay claim, that many of them think they have a Right of committing the most enormous Indecencies. And what renders them still more intolerable, is, that they never make Allowance for juvenile Extravagance, or youthful Gaiety. An old Fellow believes that his Age gives a Credit and Sanction to every Thing he says. He sits in his Elbow Chair, with a sagacious Pipe in his Mouth, interrogates magisterially concerning other People's Business, asserts with Boldness, and knocks you down with a Whiff or a F——, if you ask for an Argument ... If Men were always good and Virtuous, in Proportion to their Years, how beautiful wou'd be the Appearance of grey Hairs . . .

Centenarians, under the circumstances prevailing in the eighteenth century, were so rare that they were liable to attract almost as much attention as television stars and pop singers do today. Some who claimed to have lived to 105 years or more have been shown, since, to have been impostors, or merely mistaken, but others whose longevity was noticed by the *Gentleman's Magazine* and other news-carrying periodicals were almost certainly genuinely reported—Mrs Bailey of Liverpool, for instance, who died in 1786 aged 105 (she 'retained the perfect use of all her senses to the last; never took medicine nor was bled thro' the whole course of her life, and could see to read perfectly well without spectacles') or Mrs Boston, of the alms-house at Temple Balsall, Warwickshire, who, a few months before her death which took place in 1783 at the age of 109 years, was 'so hale as to be able to walk 2 miles, which she performed for pleasure of seeing some of her grandchildren'. How true, one wonders, was the report (in the *Gentleman's Magazine* of August 1733) of the decease of one unusually long-lived cleric?

> . . . At *Guarda* in *Portugal*, one Father *Antonio Sequiera D'Albuquerque*, who had been 86 Years Canon of the Cathedral Church, in *May* last, when he was 114 Years old, cut an entire new Set of Teeth, small, regular, and white as Ivory: His long, white Beard turn'd black, as did his Eye-brows, and the Hair on his Head. He had retain'd the perfect use of his Senses; his Nerves, relax'd by Age, began to contract, and his Muscles seemed filling out with a Juvenile Robustness; when a Fever seizing him, he died . . .

Long before the eighteenth century started, wise men had been trying to find a simple but sure method of lengthening human life. Most—if not all—of these savants had pondered in vain, but the teachings of a few of them were still influencing medical thought, and human behaviour, during the period under review.

There were the principles enunciated by Luigi Cornaro the Venetian, for instance. In the *Spectator* of 13 October 1711, Joseph

Addison wrote in praise of a little book compiled by Cornaro which had been first published at Padua in the year 1558, and had been translated into English under the title *A Sure and Certain Method of Attaining a Long and Healthy Life*. The author, said Addison, had been of an infirm constitution until he had reached the fairly advanced age of forty years. Then, by obstinately persisting in an 'exact course of temperance'—dieting strictly, and allowing himself only minute quantities of wine—he had recovered a perfect state of health. When he reached eighty, and was still as sound as a bell, the Venetian had celebrated the prolonged mellow autumn of his years by producing his famous booklet. He lived to see at least three more editions of his great work through the press. Then, having passed his hundredth year, he died 'without pain or agony and like one who falls asleep'. Cornaro's treatise, concluded Addison, had been written 'with such a spirit of cheerfulness, religion, and good sense, as are the natural concomitants of temperance and sobriety'.

Francis Bacon's cautionary precepts were still being repeated, too, in the eighteenth century.

Bacon, who was born in 1561 and who died in 1621, firmly believed that the sentiments the parents feel for each other at the very moment of conception can powerfully affect the resulting infant's expectation of life. Excessive heat of passion in the parent's sexual relations would spoil a child's prospects of longevity, he considered. Life within man being a subtle flame that feeds on some volatile 'spirits', argued Bacon, 'alacrity in the generation' would beget 'lusty and lively children', but would be 'less profitable to long life because of the acrimony and inflaming of the "spirits"'.

Almost at the very end of the eighteenth century—in 1796, to be precise—one of the most notorious of all the so-called 'experts' on longevity published his *magnum opus*. This was the versatile and philanthropic Christian Wilhelm Hufeland, of Langensalza in Prussia, who was professor at the time at Jena, and who was thirty-five years of age only when his treatise on the art of lengthening life—the *Makrobiotik*—first appeared in print. In spite of Doctor Hufeland's skill at exposing other people's fallacies—he worked hard to correct popular misconceptions about Brunonianism, Mesmerism, and other fashionable fancies—

many of the instructions given in his book appear now to be the merest nonsense. (He warned people who had dark complexions and dark hair against all animal food, for instance, but he allowed fair people to eat as much of it as they liked.) The unreliable nature of the author's recommendations would seem to be borne out by the fact that he, himself, managed to live only to the age of seventy-three, expiring after a long and agonizing illness which necessitated a delicate surgical operation performed without an anaesthetic. According to Doctor F L Augustine, who was Hufeland's biographer, a post-mortem held on the unfortunate author revealed that the patient had been suffering from a diseased prostatic gland, with an almost complete stoppage of the urethra.

Throughout history, middle-aged men and women have wanted to become young once again, and the old have wished to return, if possible, to the lesser discomforts of middle age. By the year 1700, rejuvenation had become a popular subject of controversy, and a number of medical men were vying with each other in their attempts to solve, once and for all, the problems of senescence and decline.

One of the most sensational of the eighteenth-century rejuvenators—the German physician Doctor J H Cohausen, who was born in 1665—was a man of some literary ability with a very vivid imagination. In 1742 Cohausen published his extraordinary work *Hermippus Redivivus, or the Sage's Triumph over Old Age and the Grave*. In this book, the doctor claimed that he had discovered an entirely successful method of rejuvenating people who were advanced in years. The recipe came, he said, from an ancient gravestone that had been found in or near Rome. This message was carved on the stone:

> Aesculapio et Sanitati
> L. Clodius Hermippus
> Qui vixit annos CXV Dies V
>   Puellarum anhelitu
> Quod etiam post mortem ejus
> Non Parum mirantur Physici
> Jam Posteri sic Vitam Ducite

As translated and interpreted by Doctor Cohausen, the inscription recorded the fact that 'one Hermippus, said to have lived 115 years' never grew old, having been rejuvenated by inhaling the breath of young girls. The doctor explained that Hermippus had evidently kept a boarding school for female pupils. Having arranged to be in their company by day and by night, the wise Roman had clearly profited from the revivifying properties of his scholars' exhalations.

Many physicians in the nineteenth century as well as in the eighteenth believed Doctor Cohausen's account of Hermippus' feat or, at least, thought it highly probable. They knew, for a start, from their Bibles that King David, when moribund, had had Abishag the Shulamite, a 'fair damsel', laid by his side 'that he might be revived by the warmth of her body'. Most of them knew, too, that the English friar Roger Bacon, who had lived during the thirteenth century, had recommended the same method for reviving wizened old individuals, though, being a monk, Bacon had had to couch his salacious advice in relatively discreet terms. Even the great expert on longevity, Doctor Hufeland, accepted the Hermippus story without serious question, pointing out that Hermann Boerhaave, the famous Leyden physician, had ventured to place a healthy youth on each side of an aged Burgomaster of Amsterdam who was critically ill—with results that had not been revealed. The story of Hermippus and his college for young ladies was not publicly shown to be false until 1931, when a Doctor H Paal published a scholarly monograph on the subject demonstrating that there had never been such a stone, and that Cohausen had invented the tale from beginning to end.

Throughout the Middle Ages, enterprising tradesmen had taken advantage of the simplicity and ignorance of their potential customers by offering preparations that would, they asserted, restore youthfulness. Usually, these false elixirs were marketed with some boastful claim that would seem to enhance their value —the 'medicine' had been concocted according to the secret recipe of some celebrated alchemist, for example, or had been used by the king himself. The trade in these spurious rejuvenators continued unabated through the whole of the eighteenth century.

The most glamorous rejuvenators sold then, and earlier, were undoubtedly those that were said to rely for their effect on the enormous power of gold. The possession of this precious metal in quantities was universally seen to confer the most exceptional privileges. It was easy, in consequence, to persuade unsophisticated people that gold introduced into the human body could produce transformations that were little short of miraculous. In his book *Myrothecium Spagiricum*, published in the seventeenth century, the French doctor P J Faber had added a pseudo-scientific gloss to this highly debatable doctrine. Gold, properly used—he said—could retard old age for a long time by strengthening the inborn heat of the body (the 'calor nativum', he called it) and by renewing the body's innate moisture (the 'humidum radicale'). With Doctor Faber's conveniently reassuring aphorisms to support their sales campaigns, dealers throughout the eighteenth century were able to charge very high prices for tiny bottles of so-called 'gold tinctures'. Understandably, these exotic potions were intended primarily for consumption by the rich, so the harm they could do was, in that respect at least, limited.

Also intended for the wealthy was the vegetable remedy sold for rejuvenating purposes in France during the eighteenth century by the mysterious Count de St Germain. The Count's remedy—according to Doctor Hufeland—consisted merely of an inexpensive infusion of sandalwood, senna leaves and fennel. But as the Count had for his patrons only the most influential people in Paris, including many members of the French Court, it seems likely that he charged a very high price for his alleged specific. Reasonably well-to-do people in Germany who required rejuvenation in the first decades of the century went to the notorious Doctor J C Dippel who recommended an animal oil—the 'Oleum Animale Dippelii'—which, he said, was distilled from the horns of stags. This oil, claimed Doctor Dippel, would lengthen human life 'by a century or two'. Doctor Dippel died in 1734 at the age of sixty-one.

People of slender means who were unable to afford gold tinctures or oils distilled from the horns of stags had to be content obviously, with more modest elixirs of life. Usually, dealers concerned with what is called today 'the lower end of the market' would offer those of their clients who wished to regain their lost youth various herbs or wild flowers from which miracle-working 'teas' might be infused. To give their wares an extra attraction, the tradesmen would generally be prepared to vouch that the blooms or grasses had been gathered at midnight when the moon was full, or on some other occasion that might be popularly supposed to be particularly auspicious. One of these cheaper herbal preparations—Kiesow's 'Elixirium ad vitam longam'— was widely distributed during the eighteenth century from Augsburg in South Germany. It was mainly compounded of aloes and other explosive natural purgatives.

In France, the most popular cheap specific sold for purposes of rejuvenation during the early part of the eighteenth century was the clear, tasteless fluid marketed under the name 'Elixir de Villars'. According to Doctor R Saundby, whose *Old Age, its Care and Treatment* was published in London in 1913, the sales of this elixir had mounted to enormous figures by 1728, but its success terminated suddenly when it was shown to consist of nothing but plain water. Indirectly, though, the Elixir de Villars may have done a notable amount of good, for the proprietor stated explicitly in his directions that while his 'preparation' was being taken, the patient would have to abstain entirely from any liquid that contained alcohol.

One of the many strange, esoteric practices that lingered on from the Middle Ages into the eighteenth century concerned rejuvenation. Since the earliest days of medicine, men and women had been observing vipers and other snakes shedding their skins, and they had come to believe that when this happened the snakes were rejuvenating themselves. From that, an obvious conclusion was erroneously reached: the flesh of vipers must contain a substance, or some substances, that would help to rejuvenate human beings. So, people intent on regaining their lost youth were often recommended to consume the flesh of vipers—or, if they preferred, to live for weeks on end on a diet of chickens that had been fed on minced snake. Even the eggs laid by viper-fed birds were almost universally assumed to possess rejuvenating virtues.

Blood transfusion—the practice which, in our present century, saves so many lives each year—was probably tried for the very first time in some vain attempt to rejuvenate an ageing patient. Certainly, during the Middle Ages, many people believed that witches who were anxious to gain new leases of life were in the habit of attacking children, and of drinking their blood. In 1492 a Jewish physician in Rome is said to have performed the operation for the benefit of the ailing Pope Innocent VIII, three boys being sacrificed by being bled to death on behalf of the aged pontiff. The sixteenth-century physician Marcilio Ficino is known to have issued serious and detailed instructions about the use of blood transfusion for the purposes of rejuvenation. He advised that the old people who wanted to become young again should imbibe the blood of young people 'in the manner of leeches' from the freshly-opened veins of any suitable donor or donors who might be willing to submit to the operation. If any elderly patient were not over-pleased at the idea of acting as a vampire in this way, said Ficino, he, or she, should be offered, instead, youthful blood that had been drawn off into a goblet and then mixed with sweetened wine.

By the beginning of the eighteenth century, when one might have expected a fair number of experiments in the field of blood transfusion to be happily in progress—William Harvey having published some seventy-two years before his conclusions that the movement of the blood in the body is continuous, and in a demonstrable cycle or circle—the whole subject was in a state of hush.

The cause of this shocked silence was a series of legal bans on blood transfusion. Not so very long before, Samuel Pepys had been describing appreciatively in his diaries the wonderful experiments conducted by one Richard Lower, a Cornish physician and physiologist, who had managed by using quills to convey the blood from the artery of one dog to the veins of another and, some two years later, had successfully introduced the blood of a lamb into the system of a healthy but mildly insane young man. Then, in Paris, Jean Baptiste Denis, physician to Louis XIV, had conducted some similar operations but, unfortunately, one of his human patients had died. Denis had been charged with murder. After a prolonged battle in the courts, the unlucky doctor had been exonerated, but both he and the practice of blood transfusion had been declared to be criminal by the Faculty of Medicine in Paris and had been proscribed, supposedly for ever. The English parliament had soon afterwards also declared the operation illegal, and the magistrates at Rome had quickly followed the examples of their French and English contemporaries. Interest in the possibilities offered by the transfusion of blood was quashed, therefore, during almost the whole of the period with which this book is mainly to deal.

It was roused, temporarily, just before the eighteenth century ended, when the energetic and enterprising Doctor Erasmus Darwin, grandfather of the great Charles, published his book *Zoonomia*, which contained this stimulating passage:

... Above thirty years ago I proposed to an old gentleman, whose throat was entirely impervious, to supply him with a few ounces of blood daily from an ass, or from the human animal, who is still more patient and tractable, in the following manner. To fix a silver pipe about an inch long to each extremity of a chicken's gut, the part between the two silver ends to be measured by filling it with warm water; to put one end into the vein of a person hired for that purpose, so as to receive the blood returning from the extremity; and when the gut was quite full, and the blood running through the other silver end, to introduce that end into the vein of the patient upwards towards the heart, so as to admit no air along with the blood. And, lastly, to support the gut and silver ends on a water plate, filled with water of ninety-eight degrees of heat, and to measure how many ounces of blood was introduced by passing the finger, so as to compress the gut, from the receiving pipe to the delivering pipe; and thence to determine how many gut-fills were given from the healthy person to the patient. Mr ——— considered a day on this proposal, and then another day, and at length answered, that 'he now found himself near the house of death; and that if he could return, he was now too old to have much enjoyment of life; and therefore he wished rather to proceed to the end of that journey, which he was now so near, and which he must at all events soon go, than return for so short a time'. He lived but a few days afterwards, and seemed quite careless and easy about the matter ...

After a brief flurry, interest in the subject was again allowed to lapse.

There is a story—almost certainly apochryphal—about Benjamin Franklin and his attitude to old age and death. When Franklin, according to this improbable legend, was in France, he received from America a quantity of Madeira wine, which had been bottled in Virginia. In some of the bottles he found a few dead flies, which he exposed to the warm sun in the month of July. In less than three hours, these apparently dead creatures recovered life, which had been so long suspended. At first, the revived flies appeared as if convulsed. They then raised themselves on their legs, washed their eyes with their fore feet, dressed their wings with those behind, and began in a little time to fly about. The acute philosopher proposed, therefore, the following question: 'Since, by such a complete suspension of all internal as well as external consumption, it is possible to produce a pause of life and at the same time to preserve the vital principle, might not such a process be employed in regard to man? And if that be the case,' he is said to have added, like a true patriot, 'I can imagine no greater pleasure than to cause myself to be immersed along with a few good friends in Madeira wine, and to be again called to life at the end of fifty or more years, by the genial solar rays of my native country, only that I may see what improvement the state has made, and what changes time has brought along with it.'

Had Franklin in fact been preserved in good old Madeira wine with a few of his friends, he and they, if brought to life again like the flies but in the twentieth century, would certainly be mightily surprised by the strides that have been made since their time in the practice of medicine and surgery. To him, and them, the changes made in the past two centuries—in these fields, if in no other— would seem little short of miraculous. 'Be thankful that you are alive in the twentieth century!' they would probably urge anyone who would slow down sufficiently to listen to them. 'You don't know how lucky you are!'

So, this sad review of the art of healing in the eighteenth century ought not to end on a note of regret, but with a sense of enjoyment and relief. Let it conclude, then, with part of one more item of news from the *Gentleman's Magazine*—an obituary notice this time, appropriately enough, from the issue dated May 1733. It concerned a Mr John Underwood, of Whittlesea in Cambridgeshire:

... At his Burial, when the Service was over, an Arch was turn'd over the Coffin, in which was placed a small piece of white Marble, with this Inscription, *Non omnis moriar,* 1733. Then the 6 Gentlemen who follow'd him to the Grave sung the last Stanza of the 20th Ode of the 2d Book of *Horace.* No Bell was toll'd, no one invited but the 6 Gentlemen, and no Relation follow'd his Corpse; the Coffin was painted Green, and he laid in it with all his Cloaths on; under his Head was placed *Sanadon's Horace,* at his feet *Bentley's* Milton; in his Right Hand a small Greek Testament ... After the Ceremony was over they went back to his House, where his Sister had provided a cold Supper; the Cloth being taken away the Gentlemen sung the 31st Ode of the 1st Book of *Horace,* drank a chearful Glass, and went Home about Eight. He left near 6000 l. to his Sister, on Condition of her observing this his Will, order'd her to give each of the Gentlemen ten Guineas, and desir'd they would not come in black Cloaths; The Will ends thus—*Which done I would have them take a chearful Glass, and think no more of* John Underwood ...

Select Bibliography

As well as the books and pamphlets mentioned in the text, these are the works that have been principally consulted:

ACKERKNECHT, ERWIN H. *A Short History of Medicine*. Ronald Press Co, New York, 1955

ADDISON, WILLIAM. *English Spas*. B T Batsford Ltd, London, 1951

ASHBURN, P M. *A History of the Medical Department of the United States Army*. Houghton Mifflin Company, Boston and New York, 1929

AVELING, J H, MD, FSA. *The Chamberlens and the Midwifery Forceps*. J and A Churchill, London, 1882

BERDOE, EDWARD, LRCP, MRCS. *The Origin and Growth of the Healing Art*. Swan Sonnenschein and Company, London, 1893

BISHOP, W J. *The Early History of Surgery*. Robert Hale Limited, London, 1960

BLOMFIELD, J, OBE, MD. *St George's 1733–1933*. The Medici Society, London, 1933

BUCK, ALBERT H, BA, MD. *The Growth of Medicine from the Earliest Times to about 1800*. Oxford University Press, London, 1917

CLENDENING, LOGAN, MD. *Source Book of Medical History*. Paul B Hoeber, Inc, New York, 1942

CRAWFURD, RAYMOND, MA, MD Oxon, FRCP. *The King's Evil*. The Clarendon Press, Oxford, 1911

DE ROPP, ROBERT S. *Man Against Ageing*. Victor Gollancz Limited, London, 1961

DUDLEY, T B. *A Complete History of Royal Leamington Spa*. P and W E Linaker, Leamington, 1901

ERNEST, MAURICE, LL D. *The Longer Life*. Adam and Co, London (After 1931)

FRENCH, BRIGADIER C N, CMG, CBE. *The Story of St Luke's Hospital*. William Heinemann, London, 1951

FRIEDMAN, REUBEN, MD. *The Story of Scabies.* Froben Press Inc, New York, 1947

GARRISON, FIELDING H, AB, MD. *An Introduction to the History of Medicine.* W B Saunders Company, Philadelphia and London, 1913

GARRISON, FIELDING H, AB, MD. *History of Medicine.* W B Saunders Company, Philadelphia and London, 1929

GRANVILLE, J MORTIMER, MD, FSS. *The Care and Cure of the Insane.* Hardwicke and Bogue, London, 1877

GUTHRIE, DOUGLAS, MD, FRCS (ED), FRSE. *A History of Medicine.* Thomas Nelson and Sons Ltd, London, 1945

HART, GWEN. *A History of Cheltenham.* Leicester University Press, Leicester, 1965

HOLBROOK, STEWART H. *The Golden Age of Quackery.* The Macmillan Company, New York, 1959

JAMESON, ERIC. *The Natural History of Quackery.* Michael Joseph, London, 1961

JONES, KATHLEEN, PH D. *Lunacy, Law and Conscience 1744–1845.* Routledge and Kegan Paul, London, 1955

LAFFIN, JOHN. *Surgeons in the Field.* Edward Dent, London, 1970

LAWRENCE, R M. *Primitive Psycho-Therapy and Quackery.* Constable and Company, London, 1910

LEE, EDWIN. *The Baths of Germany (Second Edition).* Whittaker and Company, London, 1843

LLOYD, CHRISTOPHER, FR HIST S, and JACK L S COULTER, FRCS. *Medicine and The Navy 1200–1900*, Volume III. E and S Livingstone Ltd, Edinburgh and London, 1961

MACPHERSON, JOHN, MD. *The Baths and Wells of Europe.* Edward Stanford, London, 1888

METCHNIKOFF, ÉLIE (translated by P Chalmers Mitchell, MA). *The Prolongation of Life.* William Heinemann, London, 1907

METTLER, CECILIA C. *History of Medicine.* The Blakiston Company, Philadelphia and Toronto, 1947

NORBURN, A E, MD, and others. *The Book of Bath. Written for the Ninety-third Annual Meeting of the British Medical Association held at Bath in July 1925.* Published at Bath

O'DONOGHUE, E G. *The Story of Bethlehem Hospital from its Foundation in 1247.* T Fisher Unwin, London, 1914

PARSONS, F G, DSC, FRCS, FSA. *The History of St Thomas's Hospital.* Methuen and Company, London, 1934

RUHRÄH, JOHN, MD. *Pædiatrics of the Past.* Paul B Hoeber, Inc, New York, 1925

SMITH, BRIAN S. *A History of Malvern.* Leicester University Press, Leicester, 1964

SPENCER, HERBERT R, MD, BS Lond. *The History of British Midwifery from 1650 to 1800.* John Bale, Sons and Danielsson Limited, London, 1927

STILL, GEORGE FREDERIC, MA, MD, HON LL D, FRCP. *The History of Paediatrics.* Oxford University Press, London, 1931

TEBB, W SCOTT, MA, MD, DPH. *A Century of Vaccination.* Swan Sonnenschein and Company, London, 1899

THOMPSON, C J S. *The Quacks of Old London.* Brentano's Limited, London, 1928

THOMS, WILLIAM J, FSA. *Human Longevity, Its Facts and its Fictions,* John Murray, London, 1873

TUKE, D HACK, MD, LL D. *The Insane in the United States and Canada.* H K Lewis, London, 1885

WALKER, KENNETH, MA, MB, FRCS. *The Story of Medicine.* Hutchinson and Company, London, 1954

Index